W9-AQF-093

Fairmount   Nov 2018

This item no longer
belongs to Davenport
Public Library

FRIENDS
of the
Davenport Public Library

"Celebrate The Printed Word"
Endowment Fund
provided funds for the
purchase of this item

Bad Advice

DAVENPORT PUBLIC LIBRARY
321 MAIN STREET
DAVENPORT, IOWA 52801-1490

Bad Advice

How to Survive and Thrive in an Age of Bullshit

DR. VENUS NICOLINO

PAUL FELDMAN, CO-WRITER

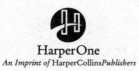

HarperOne
An Imprint of HarperCollinsPublishers

HarperOne

BAD ADVICE. Copyright © 2018 by Venus Nicolino. All rights reserved. Printed in the United States of America. No part of this book may be used or reproduced in any manner whatsoever without written permission except in the case of brief quotations embodied in critical articles and reviews. For information, address HarperCollins Publishers, 195 Broadway, New York, NY 10007.

HarperCollins books may be purchased for educational, business, or sales promotional use. For information, please email the Special Markets Department at SPsales@harpercollins.com.

FIRST EDITION

Designed by Ad Librum

Library of Congress Cataloging-in-Publication Data

Names: Nicolino, Venus.
Title: Bad advice : how to survive and thrive in an age of bullshit / Venus Nicolino.
Description: First edition. | New York, NY : HarperOne, [2018] | Includes bibliographical references.
Identifiers: LCCN 2018032071 (print) | LCCN 2018035063 (ebook) | ISBN 9780062570383 (e-book) | ISBN 9780062570352 (hardcover)
Subjects: LCSH: Self-actualization (Psychology) | Self-realization. | Self-perception. | Conduct of life.
Classification: LCC BF637.S4 (ebook) | LCC BF637.S4 N525 2018 (print) | DDC 158.1—dc23
LC record available at https://lccn.loc.gov/2018032071

18 19 20 21 22   LSC   10 9 8 7 6 5 4 3 2 1

This book is dedicated to the person who was on my mind the most while I was writing it. YOU.

CONTENTS

WHY ARE YOU READING THIS?

Let's be real before you read any further:

The premise of this book is fucked.

This is a self-help book. The *self* in question is you, and the one doing the helping is me. I've got some nerve, huh? Without ever knowing a single thing about you or even meeting you, I'm going to give you tools and techniques to know yourself better, cope with whatever shit life throws at you, and get more out of being alive than you ever thought possible. *That's* the fucked premise we're going with here. And I gotta say . . . it sounds super dumb. But that dumb process and fucked premise aren't unique to this book: They're the backbone of the entire self-help genre. Then what makes this book different? Why isn't *this* self-help book fucked and dumb? Because I didn't write it under the assumption that *you* are either fucked or dumb.

First off, you are now reading a self-help book called *Bad Advice*. That tells me you've got an edgy sense of humor and you're not into the usual saccharine, sanctimonious bullshit that passes for self-help. (I hate that shit, too. OMG we have so much in common already! Why aren't we following each other on Insta!?) The fact that you're reading a self-help book tells me something else: You know that life ain't always easy-peasey-lemon-squeezey. Life can sting, burn, and cut like a motherfucker. Pain comes in no shortage of flavors—heartbreak, loneliness, loss, disappointment, and frustration to name some of the Greatest Hits. Life can be scary. It's full of things that are unknown, out of your control, or both. Once you've gone through enough pain, you quickly discover that all that great, wise-sounding self-help advice doesn't help for shit. It doesn't help because it's *Bad Advice*. It never helped you cope. It never eased your pain. It never truly inspired you. Ya know why? Because it's not inspiration. It's bullshit. It's #BadAdvice. And because it never works, #BadAdvice never leaves you feeling better. At its root, all #BadAdvice operates off the same flawed theory: *Emotions are optional. So when you feel bad, it's not only your choice: It's your fault.*

How do you know #BadAdvice when you hear it? Check out a few specimens of #BadAdvice I collected in the field. Like this one: *You Can't Love Anyone Until You Love Yourself.* Sure you can. Self-hate never stopped anyone from falling in love. *Nobody Can Make You Feel Bad Without Your Permission.* When was the exact moment you gave someone permission to hurt your feelings? (Hint: Never.) *Expectations Lead to Disappointment.* For fuck's sake, THAT #BADADVICE IS A GODDAMN EXPECTATION. People create #BadAdvice when they confuse deep-sounding fluff with something wise and inspirational. I can't blame anyone for trying to get #BadAdvice to work. Easing pain is a natural, healthy instinct. The problem is, #BadAdvice doesn't ease your pain: It tries to deny your pain out of existence.

Still, you gotta do *something* when the emotional shit hits the situational fan. It's why you picked up this book. So huddle up: This very moment you're in right now, reading these words, marks the Beginning of Something Big for you. (I'm stoked I can be here for it.) I know it's the start of something big because again, you're seeking help from a book called *Bad Advice*. To me, that says that something at your core is already telling you those flowery phrases and the ideas behind them are bullshit. But there's actually some good in all that #BadAdvice, because it inspired you to seek out something better. Your search is what brought us together here, right now in this moment. From here we go on together. And you should know that I've got your back.

You're about to get a shitload of #GoodAdvice. When you finish this book, you'll be ready to do more than "get the most you can out of life": You'll be empowered *to get the most you can out of you*. Shit, let's get the most we can out of this book: We're not even all the way through the Introduction and I already have some #GoodAdvice for you, in the form of a question: *What if you already have everything you need?* What if the reason it feels like there's no way out of your problems is because you have your back to the exit? What if most of what this society—and by extension your teachers, friends, family, or even therapists—has told you about yourself *isn't true*? What if the culture you live in doesn't understand human emotions or how to engage them? What if everything you've learned about what it means to be happy and successful is wrong?

#GoodAdvice is not a prescription for pain-free living. Only #BadAdvice makes that impossible promise. But #GoodAdvice *can* help you tap into strengths, talents, and potential that are already within you, waiting to be discovered. My #GoodAdvice does not provide you with any Capital-A Answers to Life's Big Questions. It wouldn't be #GoodAdvice if it did. When you act on #GoodAdvice, *you* are the one finding the answers to the Big Questions. That's a big deal, because you are the only person in the world qualified to do that for yourself.

I'm not gonna lie: It's inevitable that life will sometimes hurt and/or scare the shit out of you. *But sometimes life is fucking flat-out fantastic.* It can fill you with joy, laughter, and a gabillion other flavors of pleasure: Your favorite song. The Grand Canyon. Orgasms. Waking up in the morning. Holding/being held by the one you love. Netflix. And all you have to do is just *be,* and you automatically earn a lifetime front row seat to all of that. Your emotions are not your enemies. They're not useless. They're not obstacles. And they sure as shit aren't meaningless. They are internal messengers we evolved to help us survive and interact with the world around us, and *there is no opt-out feature.* So what you need to do is learn the best way for you to opt in to *all* your emotions—good, bad, and everywhere in between.

So even though I don't know you, I do know why you're reading this book. You're reading this book because you're ready. You're reading this book because you want to opt in. You're reading this book because after searching for so, so long, you've finally found some #GoodAdvice.

1

JUST BE YOURSELF

How can I ace this job interview?

JUST BE YOURSELF!

Fuck. Another first date. I hate first dates. What if he doesn't like me?

JUST BE YOURSELF!

What if I bomb my presentation and I look like a total jackass?

JUST BE YOURSELF!

It's a near-guarantee that you will hear this #BadAdvice to *Just Be Yourself* at the absolute *worst* possible times. *Just Be Yourself* is the #BadAdvice you hear when you're grappling with self-doubt or the fear of rejection. It's supposed to be a confidence booster and remind you of how tremendously, indisputably *grrrrrrreat* you really are! (Cue theme from *Rocky*, or Epic Training Montage music of your choice.) But when your friend, your mom, or your favorite TV shrink tells you with the best intentions to *Just Be Yourself*, you're already being yourself. It just so happens that in that moment, the "yourself" you are being is a crazed lunatic suffering a sudden assault of the terror-shits. (That's *myself* when I'm nervous. And with that, you're now in my poop confidence. We are forever tied. This stays here). The existential panic I'm describing is set off by a systemic breakdown in your psyche. The circuit of your self-confidence shorted out because it was overloaded with confusion and self-doubt. This #BadAdvice makes it seem like you can reset your self-confidence the same way you'd flip a switch: by "just" doing it. *Just Be Yourself* sounds like an assertive directive, so we think it's strong medicine. But in reality, *Just Be Yourself* is some weak-ass sauce.

First off, this #BadAdvice uses the word "just" as an adverb. This cuts the balls off of any sentence it's in: *Just wanted to follow up* . . . *Just making sure you have that fifty bucks you owe me* . . . *Just be yourself.* It's an attempt to make the deliberate appear spontaneous. "Oh, I *just* so happened to remember it's been six months since I loaned you that fifty bucks." And you should *just so happen* to *be yourself.* As if the ongoing and involuntary action of you being you takes up the same psychological bandwidth as remembering your phone charger on your way out the door.

The #BadAdvice of *Just Be Yourself* is a mindfuck because it assumes that up until now, you've been someone other than yourself. Huh? *If this isn't me, then who am I? Who are you? What the fuck is going on? Is this #BadAdvice or #BadWeed? Just Be Yourself* is #BadAdvice because it tells you to do what you are already doing. From your first breath to your last, *you are being yourself,* with zero breaks and zero effort. Trying to *Just Be Yourself* is like trying to be deliberate about the individual beats of your heart. You can't do it.

Someone Else's Definition of Who You Are Doesn't Have to Be Your Definition

Just Be Yourself *might* be #GoodAdvice if society were ready to unconditionally accept you. But that's not the case. The society you live in has a nasty habit of defining people by a single characteristic, and conditioning *you* to define yourself by that single characteristic. It's a perception often polluted by bigotry, sexism, racism, and other small-minded, destructive bullshit.

It's why the same culture that trumpets *Age Is Just a Number* had a media shame-orgy over Madonna's fifty-eight-year-old hand. It's why in the same country where *Love Your Body* is a viral meme, eight million people struggle with eating disorders. It's why, even though we truly mean it when we say *It Gets Better,* LGBTQIA kids remain at greater risk of suicide. Your gender, race, age, sexual orientation, weight, career, socioeconomic status, or whatever else can definitely *inform* your identity, but none of them, together or alone, truly define all of who you are. *You* define who you are, but not until you ditch the #BadAdvice that tells you to *Just Be Your (Old/Fat-Ass/Faggot/Slutty/Broke-Ass) Self.*

A Claim of "I Don't Care What Anyone Thinks" Is Actually a Confession of "I Want Everyone to Think I Don't Care"

The destructive small-mindedness described above often creates a backlash. That backlash can be a very good thing. It has given us things like feminism, the civil rights movement, and legal weed. But that backlash creates other consequences. Because it's still all too easy to get hooked into the #BadAdvice to *Just Be Yourself.* Only now, the #BadAdvice is disguised as the #BadMotto of *I Don't Care What Anyone Else Thinks.* Have you ever felt this way? I know I have. Maybe you feel like this now: *I'm just gonna be myself and do what I want. I Don't Care What Anyone Else Thinks.* Why wouldn't you feel this way? How could you not be pissed off when the equation you're given for Being Yourself is this:

(You ÷ Just Be Yourself) + Who You're Told to Be = 💩

So the meta-message you receive year after year is *Just Be Yourself, You Worthless Piece of Shit.* How could you not have a knee-jerk response of *Oh yeah? We'll fuck all y'all, I'm gonna do MY thing!* You're not *Just Being Yourself* if you define your-self only by what you are not: *You're Just Being Your Anger.*

What I've found especially crazy-making is that so much of self-help culture encourages this thinking, believing it to be an expression of individualism when it's really a cry for help. And if you *really* didn't care what anyone else thought, you wouldn't need those anyones to know you didn't care. Besides, you'd have all the charisma of a parking ticket if you *really* didn't care what anyone else thought of you.

There's No Such Thing as "Self-Help": Somebody Wrote the Book, Taught the Class, Gave the Speech; Nobody Gets Through Life Alone

Another thing that makes *Just Be Yourself* #BadAdvice is the fact that you're never really by yourself. You don't operate in a vacuum. Who you are is a combination of many different things, including how you relate to and connect with other people. But let's be clear: What anyone thinks of your hair, your clothes, your skin color, your status, your sexuality, your car, your job, your gender—NONE OF THAT MATTERS. But are you a good friend? Can you be trusted? Are you kind? Are you dependable? Your words and actions send out a broad-cast of negative or positive energy that ripples far beyond the people you know. What other people think *should* matter to you, when it's your words or actions inspiring their thoughts. That's power.

Your self-awareness is the measure of how responsible you are with this power. Are you self-aware? Do you want to be? Being able to answer these questions makes the difference between spinning your wheels trying to *Just Be Yourself* and *Deciding to Know Yourself.* Self-awareness matters in the real world.

Dr. Robert S. Rubin is an award-winning professor and scholar specializing in organizational behavior. I was lucky enough to get a chance to discuss self-awareness with him, and he told me that his research found that people who were less self-aware than others "are less successful in the workplace. They don't know what they're doing *and lack the insight to know they don't know what they're doing.*" Does that sound like you? How would you even know if you're not very self-aware to begin with? This isn't an unchangeable state you have to surrender to, however. Self-knowledge and self-awareness *will* follow if instead of trying to *Just Be Yourself,* you begin to *know the self you're being.* (Deep, man.)

Self-Awareness and Self-Knowledge: Both Are a State of Being, a Decision, and a Responsibility

It's way too easy to go down a psychological black hole trying to get your head around things like self-awareness and self-knowledge. (I sure as hell did in the first draft of this chapter!) As concepts, they overlap with that heady philosophical question of *Who Am I?* Philosophers have struggled to answer that question for as long as philosophy's been a thing. But you and I don't have the time to disappear up our own asses talking about this shit, so let's keep it simple: Self-knowledge is an understanding of who you are. Self-awareness is an understanding of *why* you are who you are. You don't have to be a Plato or a Descartes to pull either of these off. And you're not starting from zero here: Recognizing that you may not know who you are and that you're always changing is in itself self-awareness. And by the way, *everybody* needs help figuring this shit out at some point. Which is why it's my mission to replace the #BadAdvice of *Just Be Yourself* with some get-real #GoodAdvice.

Go Fuck Yourself #GOODADVICE

Here's the deal: When I say, *Go Fuck Yourself,* I don't mean this: 👆; I mean this: 🥒 .

Fuck is a hard-working, versatile word. Since the fourteenth century, *fuck* has been working around the clock to help us express our strongest feelings in countless ways. Think of all the meanings and uses offered by this simple, four-letter word. It can be a noun, a verb, an adverb, or even a fucking adjective. Through a confluence of complex historical and cultural factors, we've made the word *fuck* into a vessel for the deepest things we feel. And while the stories that *fuck* began as an acronym for *Fornication Under Consent of the King* or *For Unlawful Carnal Knowledge* are not true, they do tell us something about our cultural relationship with the word. *Fuck* is such an important word to us that we invented these bogus origin stories for it, as if it were a superhero. *We are meaning-making creatures.* Even if the stories aren't real, we *want* the word *fuck* to have a deeper meaning.

So I'm gonna provide that deeper meaning for you right now. My #GoodAdvice to *Go Fuck Yourself* is actually a guide to *Go Find Understanding, Confidence, and Knowledge in Yourself.* Collect as much information as you can because your goal is to find self-connection and intimate knowledge about YOU.

So how do you *Find Understanding, Confidence, and Knowledge?* How do you *Fuck Yourself?* When you *Go Fuck Yourself*, you treat yourself in the very same way you'd treat someone you want to fuck—someone you're infatuated with. Think of how you feel and what you do when you have a crush on someone. First of all, you stalk them on all social media outlets. You check all their online photo albums. You make friends with their friends to collect intel and get closer to the target. You have a genuine curiosity about this person. You want to know what they're thinking, what they're doing, how they're feeling at every single moment of every single day. You want to know them, because you want to fuck them. You'll go out of your way to comfort them, prove yourself trustworthy, and shore up their confidence. You'll do anything to help them feel good, because if they associate being with you with feeling good, they'll be more likely to fuck you.

When you *Go Fuck Yourself*, you need to become your own obsession in the same way you obsess over someone you want to fuck. All the things you would do to get someone to fuck you are *exactly* what you need to do for yourself: *Find Understanding, Confidence, and Knowledge.* Which means you will be armed and ready the next time uncertainty, anxiety, and self-doubt start closing in. So it is with the deepest sincerity and urgency that I tell you again, *Go Fuck Yourself.* You begin this process the same way you start learning about someone you want to fuck: Wait until dark, then go through their trash, looking for clues. I kid. Do not do that. To anyone. Ever. To *Go Fuck Yourself,* you begin with another F-word: You start by *Finding.*

You Find What You Decide to Look for (Most of the Time)

Your goal is to create and sustain self-awareness and self-knowledge, so you want to *Find* as much information as you can. But you also need to be objective in the way you gather and take in that information. Self-awareness is an ongoing process of questions, answers, and questions about the answers. Meaning, you're able to recognize and accept the truth about your negative aspects as accurately as your positive ones.

Look, I get it. Most people don't head to the self-help section looking for new ways to identify negative things about themselves. And the whole point of reading a book like this is to feel better about yourself. But how can you feel better without knowing what's making you feel worse? You'll be able to access that information when you *Find* self-objectivity. This begins with your curiosity and your ability to understand how others see you.

Robert Rubin uses the common business term "external benchmarking" in a more personal way. In the business world, external benchmarks give you information about how your business compares with others or with industry best practices. In the personal sphere, external benchmarks come in the form of information about you that you collect from other people. Taking in this information is different from viewing yourself negatively. People you know are sharing their direct experience of how your words and actions affect them—in other words, *the kind of thing you should care about*. The only way to know how others experience you is to ask them. And you'll need to be ready to accept some shit you may not want to hear about yourself.

Trust Yourself to Change Yourself

#BadAdvice and crappy self-help will tell you to ignore or dismiss that kind of negative feedback. *How else are you gonna avoid feeling icky?* Look, I don't expect you to feel stoked after confronting your imperfections. But if you deny them, you're cutting yourself off from potentially valuable information. The value of this information is based on how well you understand it. Which brings us to *Understanding*, the U in the F-U-C-K of *Go Fuck Yourself*.

The way to find understanding in the information you've collected is to *filter it for consensus and context*. Do a side-by-side comparison of everything everyone tells you about you. The traits and behaviors people consistently notice are the ones most worth your time, because they're the most consistent aspects of who you are. If everyone you talk to says you're always interrupting them mid-sentence, then that's something for you to think about. If only one person says you always interrupt them mid-sentence, it's possible that person never has anything interesting to say. (Still, mind your manners, and let them finish explaining their bullshit.) Context is also important. Someone who knows you only from work or school can know you only in that context. So you'll get the best information from people who experience you in multiple contexts, because they're familiar with more than just one version of you.

Again, you may find out some shit about yourself that you don't like. That's okay, because this isn't a stroke-job for your ego. In fact, it's better than okay—it's *great*, because when you're aware of what you do, why you do it, and how others experience you, you *understand* yourself. With that understanding comes the opportunity and the choice not to *Just Be Yourself,* but to *Change Yourself.* Make the most of this opportunity. Make the commitment to *Go Fuck Yourself.*

Yeah, I said, it. The C-word! *Commitment.* C'mon, you didn't think when I told you to go *Fuck Yourself* I meant you should hit it and quit it, did you? Of course not. You wouldn't do you like that. *This isn't a one-night stand, Baby—you're here to stay!* Honoring a commitment works on more than one level. If you commit to getting more sleep, and you go to bed earlier, TA-DA! You got more sleep.

But that's not all you're doing for yourself. When you

honor a self-commitment, you begin to create self-trust. Every promise you keep adds to more, undeniable evidence of your own competence, reliability, and honesty. This is how you'll know it's not just pillow talk when you tell yourself: *I am competent. I am reliable. I am honest.* Your commitment to finding shit out about yourself, understanding the shit you find, and changing the shit you don't like is what helps you create the third component of *Fucking Yourself: Confidence*. Ah, confidence. That thing you were told you'd find if you could *Just Be Yourself.*

Commitment Is the Anchor of Confidence

So, what are you ready to commit to? As in *right now*. What are we working toward together, you and me, page by page? Who, what, and how do you want to be when you finish reading this book? Do you want to commit to being more patient? Being a kinder person? Being less afraid? Make your decision, commit to it, and then *Make a Plan*. I know you can do this. When you're trying to fuck someone, you suddenly have a better talent for logistics than a wedding planner on Adderall. You'll sync up your waxing schedule for a good first impression and juggle all the already-existing shit on your calendars to get that Great Window of Fuck to open.

So why not use that logistical genius now? Put down on paper and in detail how you will keep your commitment. You'll feel more focused, purposeful, and determined than you ever would trying to *Just Be Yourself*. Some people call this *writing a manifesto*. In business it's called a *mission statement*. I like to think of it as *Proof You're Not Bullshitting*. When you have proof you're not bullshitting, you know you can trust yourself. You'll also begin learning more about yourself.

So figure out the details of how to actually make this happen. What do you need to do? What will you need to do it? How long will it take? Who else has done it, and what can you learn from them? You live at a time when you can access everything anyone who ever lived ever knew about everything, and all you need is a Wi-Fi password (or a neighbor with an unprotected network). When you have the information, dedicate and delegate your time. Carve it out on your calendar, set up reminders on your phone. And from the moment you make your commitment onward, *write this shit down*. If your commitment is to be less afraid, before you go to bed write down the ways you chose to be more courageous than afraid that day. Write about more than that. Write about *everything*.

Write Down What You Think, And You'll See Your Thoughts Differently

The more you write, the more you'll reveal information about you. Gathering this information will help fill in that final letter K in the F-U-C-K of *Fucking Yourself: Knowledge*. Specifically, *self-knowledge*. Knowing what you can be certain of in yourself is what gives you the courage to face uncertainty. When you truly know yourself, you're able to accurately perceive yourself. Which means that when you find yourself in a moment when your confidence begins to waver, you'll have rock-solid self-knowledge to fall back on. Don't put this off. There's no reason you can't start today. Indulge the same obsessive-bordering-on-stalkerlike curiosity in yourself that you would for someone you want to fuck.

You kinda already stalk yourself online. How much time do you waste scrolling through your Facebook feed, Snapchat'n and Instagram'n yourself, delighting at each notification of a "like," a "share," or (sweet Jesus!) a *"love"*? Don't feel bad, we all do it. Since you already keep a daily document of yourself, why not get more out of it? I mean, you could actually *Go Fuck Yourself* instead of thirsting for "likes" and followers. Why not shift that energy toward yourself? Document you for YOU. *Start keeping a daily journal and write in it every day.* I know! *Writing*—when most people won't read anything longer than 140 characters. But this isn't for most people, this is just for you.

Taking the time to reflect on your day, writing down all that happened and how you felt, supplies you with a constant, updated flow of information that feeds your self-awareness. Research shows it's actually good for your health, too. Committing to writing for just fifteen to twenty minutes daily reduces stress-related activity in the brain and can even promote speedier physical healing. And while the data suggest that you'll get the most benefit from longhand writing, I do my own journaling on my phone's notepad app. You should see the volumes of shit I've tapped out on there. There are no rules to break here. This doesn't have to feel like work any more than uploading the pic of your blackberry mojito. Don't worry about grammar or spelling (I never do—ask my editor!), just as long as what you write makes sense to you. You can make it *fun*. You can make it *meaningful*. You'll learn more about who you are in five minutes of *Just Writing Yourself* than a year of trying to *Just Be Yourself*.

Self-Doubt Is the Prerequisite to Greatness

Wait . . . whaaaa? You're still here? So even after getting to know yourself, learning to trust yourself, committing to writing about yourself, not to mention fucking yourself, you're still doubting yourself? Good. That means you're not an asshole.

I realize self-doubt can be a bitch of an emotion to deal with. It's the embryo of all #BadAdvice. It can be a sludgy kind of feeling—easy to get stuck in and hard to shake off. And sure, confidence is sexy, but would you want to fuck someone who is 100 percent self-confident all the time? That's not confidence, that's arrogance: *Before we Netflix and Chill, I want you to know I'm 100 percent confident I'll be the best you ever had, Baby. Now move over so I can see myself in the mirror.* And like every other one of your emotions, self-doubt has its uses. It can drive you to prove yourself and get shit done.

I don't have two master's degrees and a PhD because I think I'm smart. I got them because I think I'm dumb. Self-doubt is emotional booze: A little bit can put fire under your ass, but too much will leave you on the floor.

So when it comes to taking my #GoodAdvice to *Go Fuck Yourself*, the idea is to *balance*—not replace self-doubt with self-confidence. The #GoodAdvice to *Go Fuck Yourself* empowers you to be confident enough to believe in yourself but still wise enough to find the benefit in doubting yourself.

Fuck Yourself and Free Yourself

The expression to *Just Be Yourself* evolved into #BadAdvice because at some point everyone has a desperate need to ease their own self-doubt and the anxieties that go with it. But you can't merely reject #BadAdvice—you have to replace it. So are you ready? I think you are. You've waited long enough. It's time to take your relationship with you to the next level. It's time to *Go Fuck Yourself.* And like any good relationship expert, I have some #FuckTips, should you need an assist with *Fucking Yourself.* So here goes.

Don't Underestimate Your Selfie's Worth

Don't just *Go Fuck Yourself, Go Fuck Your Selfie.* That's right, I'm appropriating another fuck-conjugation, and I'm doing so with science, mofos. A University of California, Irvine, research team found that college students who regularly took selfies and shared them with others showed an increase in feelings of confidence and self-acceptance. So it can be #GoodAdvice to *Just See Yourself.* It's also worth mentioning that the students were specifically told to smile in their selfies.

Now look, I get that nobody likes being told to smile, especially when your emotional state feels like the opposite of a smile. Women have to put up with this shit all the time. (Like when I'm walking down the street and some jackass yells, "Smile pretty lady!" *Silly me! I forgot that my purpose in life is to provide entertainment for strangers on benches.*) What makes my suggestion to smile in your selfie different is that it has to come from your decision to lift your mood and confidence, and the science on smiling is pretty compelling. Researchers have found that smiling can lower your heart rate and stress levels. The physical act of smiling also appears to trigger happy memories, which can offer an emotional boost. Even people who had their mouths physically forced into a smile by holding a pencil or chopsticks between their teeth exhibited some of these benefits. So don't just selfie; selfie and *smile.* (And smile for real . . . no duck lips.)

The Music That Made You Feel Bulletproof as a Kid Can Do the Same Thing Now

Nothing sets the mood for fucking quite like music, so get started on making that proverbial mix tape for yourself. There's a reason stadiums full of sports fans still get psyched up when they clap and stamp along to Queen's *We Will Rock You* (aside from it being a kick-ass song). Researchers have found that listening to bass heavy music can make you feel powerful and confident. They explain this effect with what they call the "contagion hypothesis": The emotions in the music you listen to can shape the emotions you feel. Ever been brought to tears in the middle of a great day by a sad song? Scientists believe that since our culture associates low, bass-heavy sounds with power and confidence, listening to bass-heavy music can inspire the same kinds of feelings, no matter if it's the driving rhythm of EDM or a thunderous Beethoven symphony. So if you need a power-up before you make a speech or head to the Big Meeting, grab your headphones and give yourself a quickie.

The Best Friends Still Remember Who You Are When You Forget

It's always a big moment when the person you want to fuck meets your friends. What your friends think matters to you, because you respect them. And your friends' support counts just as much when you're fucking yourself into confidence, because when someone you respect compliments you, you believe them. Some might call this a placebo effect, but "placebo" translates from Latin to *Who gives a fuck as long as it works?*

So, who are the peeps you hang with? How do you feel when you're around them? What do they help you believe about you? Can you trust them? If you're not sure, do a quick head count of the people you know who trust you. In trusting you, they've proved themselves worthy of *your* trust. You aren't responsible for how other people help you feel, but you can decide on the kind of help you want. No matter how you feel, you're going to *Just Be Yourself.* If you need to change how you feel, start looking at who you choose to be with.

Ritual: A Small Investment with a Guaranteed High Rate of Return

Data from numerous studies shows that practicing *rituals* can also boost your self-confidence. And look, if the word "ritual" makes you think of eating a dry wafer and drinking grape juice or chanting naked under a full moon, let me offer you a reframe. Our culture has all kinds of weird, complicated rituals related to fucking. Collectively, these fuck-centered rituals are called "dating." And if people don't act dumb and make dating a pain in the ass, the rituals build trust and confidence for people, all leading up to . . . you know where this is going.

To create an effective ritual for yourself, all you need is a simple, repeatable action you can use when you need to create confidence. Grab that daily journal you just started keeping and take five minutes to write about how confident you are, even if you only write the sentence *I am confident.* Find a good luck charm and make a ritual of taking it everywhere with you. Fill out that application with your lucky pen and wear your lucky socks to the job interview.

This might sound like New Age Bullshit, but there's reliable Digital Age Science that you can make your own luck when you make yourself feel lucky. In one study, golfers had better results when told they were using a "lucky ball." German researchers found that people's performance improved after being told someone had their fingers crossed for them. (They were actually told someone was "pressing the thumbs"—the German version of crossing fingers. No one has yet studied why luck is generated differently in Germany.) Fingers, thumbs, balls—it really doesn't matter. Feeling lucky comes from an inner belief, not an outer condition. You won't worry about how to *Just Be Yourself* when you can *Go Fuck Yourself* into feeling lucky.

Your Sense of Self Is Shaped by Your Senses

Fucking yourself into confidence, like fucking anyone else, is a sensuous experience. The difference is your senses feed your confidence, instead of pleasure. So when you're looking to ease self-doubt, you'd do better to *Just Smell Yourself* over trying to *Just Be Yourself.* And don't worry if you're fresh out of the gym with smelly pits; I'm not talking about your own musk. Studies have found that whether you're a man or a woman, wearing a fragrance you're especially fond of can increase your self-confidence. Not only that, but your confidence will grow in proportion to how much you like the scent you're wearing. In other words, it's possible for your sense of smell to inform your sense of self. (Note to Marketing Department: Start developing signature perfume called *Confidence: A New Fragrance from Dr. V.*)

What You Project Colors What's Perceived

We're all in agreement that red is the official color of fucking, right? Red is sensual. It's vibrant. It's bold. It's hot. And when you're *Fucking Yourself* into confidence, you should be seeing red. Numerous studies have found that wearing the color red can help you feel more confident. But *Go Fuck Yourself Red* isn't a hue for your eyes only. Other research has shown that people wearing red are often *perceived* as being more confident. When people perceive you as confident, they'll treat you like you're confident, and that helps you *feel* confident. How much you do or don't care what anyone else thinks has nothing to do with how confident you are: It doesn't figure into the equation. Confidence doesn't happen in a vacuum. Much like love, it is a co-creation between you and other people.

You Are More than What You See.
You Are More than What Others See.
You Are More than You Know.

Just Be Yourself isn't just #BadAdvice, it's #UselessAdvice. As long as you're still breathing, you will continue to *Just Be Yourself*. And unless you're a narcissistic garbage fire of a person, there will always be times when you doubt yourself. But will you know yourself? Will you trust yourself? Will you be self-aware? My #GoodAdvice to *Go Fuck Yourself* might not make the daytime talk circuit, but it will help answer those questions.

My idea of fucking is a simultaneous expression and creation of intimacy. Intimacy is a deep, personal knowledge and understanding of someone. *Fucking Yourself* means

creating a deep, personal knowledge of *you*. Any self-help
schlep can tell you to *Just Be Yourself*, smile, and sign your
copy of their book. That's not me. I can't make you confident. Real, deep confidence results from a fusion of self-
awareness, self-knowledge, and self-trust. When you can't
access that right away, you don't need to *Just Be Yourself*,
you need to *Go Fuck Yourself*. Seduce yourself into confidence. Jedi Mind Trick yourself out of self-doubt. Feed your
heart and mind with music, colors, sweat, and scents. Trick
yourself into being confident long enough to remember all
the undeniable reasons you have to believe and trust in
yourself.

You Are More than What You See.

You Are More than What Others See.

You Are More than You Know.

So *Go Find Understanding, Confidence, and Knowledge* in
Yourself.

GO FUCK YOURSELF

#GOODADVICE

2

YOU CAN'T LOVE ANYONE UNTIL YOU LOVE YOURSELF

I'm still not 100 percent sure what love is. Are you? Do you know it when you feel it? When love shows its face, do you throw yourself at it full-bore? Do you hide? Do you tell it to fuck off? How do you love? Who do you love? Do you love yourself? *Can* you love yourself? I mean, is it really #BadAdvice to try to love yourself before you love someone else? After all, if you could you love yourself, you wouldn't have to waste energy wondering whether you *really* "like yourself in that way." You'd know whether you were seeing anyone else already, you've already met your parents, and you'd be the first to know if you fucked someone besides you. Sounds like a safer bet, no? So why not Swipe Right on yourself? (Although wait a sec . . . if you want to Swipe Right on yourself, does that mean you really need to swipe left? Fuck it, you know what I mean.) But *You Can't Love Anyone Until You Love Yourself* is not a safer bet—it's #BadAdvice. What it really tells you is this: *You're a Loser at Love Because You're Too Stupid to Love.* And *that* is some of the #WorstAdvice I've ever heard.

But it also symbolizes a crisis of our expectations of love in the modern world. It's a crisis arising from a conflict of psychology, biological desires, and social-cultural messages. And it's a crisis that can only happen in the comfort of the First World: A privileged culture promotes privileged relationships. We get nearly anything we want at the touch of a button or a Swipe Right, and we expect the same of love. But even privileged relationships fail—even when love is reduced to a depersonalized experience on par with an Amazon purchase: a Swipe Right, you buy. Unhappy with your purchase, want to return it? Ghost 'em, no questions asked.

Still, we fall in love. Hearts still break. And we have no control over or understanding of the how and why of it all. So we lie to ourselves and hide behind this #BadAdvice. We use bullshit lines like *I just didn't love myself enough* or *She just didn't love herself enough* as placeholders for real understanding, and then we try to move on. This is how too many of us learn to see love—through the disposable lens of consumerism that dictates, "Use once and destroy."

People seem to apply this #BadAdvice only to Romantic Love. No five-year-old has ever said, "Easy on the hugs, Grandma; I can't love you until I love myself." Maybe we don't apply this #BadAdvice to familial love because deep down, *everyone already suspects it's bullshit.* But then why do we keep trying to believe this is true for Romantic Love? Because this #BadAdvice makes a false promise. *You Can't Love Anyone Until You Love Yourself* promises to hide you from a specific flavor of pain: the pain of a broken heart. That's not just bullshit, it's fucking crazy: *How can you hide from something inside you?* Going along with this #BadAdvice means accepting that when it comes to Romantic Love, you exist in a state of wrongness and stupidity. What other reason could there be for your breakup, your heartache, or your feeling rejected? *You!* You're a loser at love because you don't even love yourself (insert sad emoji face).

When you first hear it, *You Can't Love Anyone Until You Love Yourself* sounds kind of truthy, because it offers comfort in something so many of us desperately want to be true— that there's an opt-out feature on heartbreak. But the truth is, when it comes to love, you're along for the ride. You will fall in and out of love. Your heart will be broken. And you have no say in how any of that goes down. *You Can't Love Anyone Until You Love Yourself* offers an illusion of control over Romantic Love. That's more than just #BadAdvice. It's a denial of reality.

Love Is Not Sequential; Love Is Synchronous

The idea of loving yourself "first" implies that love happens as a sequence of events: *First, I love me. Next, I love you.* Even without looking at any scientific data, psychological theories, or what you read a few paragraphs back, you know this is bullshit. *You are already loving people.* There's also a connotation that loving yourself "first" means loving yourself *most*: *I can't worry about her feelings, I have to love myself first.*

But Romantic Love invented the idea of equal opportunity; it has no prerequisites. Love gives not one single fuck about your plans or expectations, let alone if you love yourself. It's one of the most powerful, volatile things you can experience. Romantic Love will either get you higher than a trust-fund hippie at Coachella or tear you up worse than a victim in a *Saw* movie. And you have zero control over it. Add zero understanding of love to zero control, and you increase love's fear factor. *You Can't Love Anyone Until You Love Yourself* denies that fear. It's another variation on the same unfulfillable promise made by other #BadAdvice: *Emotions are optional.*

English philosopher and Zen scholar Alan Watts compared following this #BadAdvice to you "trying to outwit yourself." Watts said that ". . . trying to love yourself is like trying to kiss your own lips." He suggested that our cultural "rules" of love might function better as Zen koans, those nonsensical, third-eye-opening-type riddles like "What is the sound of one hand clapping?" or "What is the color of the wind?" or "You can't love anyone until you love yourself." Meditating on the impossible logic of a koan is supposed to exhaust your reasoning, leaving your mind ready to perceive deeper truths without overthinking them. Koans are not advice: They're actually #NonAdvice. Mr. Watts was onto something here. For centuries, the word "love" has fallen short of describing a thing that is indescribable: It's a feeling, a state of being, an action, and an outside force acting upon you all at once. So if we treat *You Can't Love Anyone Until You Love Yourself* as a koan, it's surprisingly helpful, because it shows us what love isn't: *a choice.*

We Are a Species of Infinite Individuality That Loves Identically

When his story begins, Harry Potter is an ordinary kid in the ordinary world who can't understand the random magic shit that happens around him. Then he discovers he has magical powers, learns to use them, and goes on to kick seven books' worth of magical ass.

Your ability to love is the same. You were born with it, and you can learn to elevate love from an automatic function to something deliberate and meaningful. You don't have to achieve some kind of inward-facing, imaginary perfection before you can love someone else. You're already doing it. Simply by being in the world, you are already loving and loved.

When you were a toddler, something in your cells pushed you to try to start walking. You fell down and got bumped and bruised while you were figuring it out, but it was something your body already knew it could do, because it's part of its design. Love is part of that physical design, too. So your body, and by extension you, is already able to love. Scientific studies have shown that being in love changes your brain. The release of the biochemicals that make you feel in love with someone are an involuntary action, and they don't care how you feel about yourself. Don't believe me? Don't worry. Your biology will outwit your psychology.

Dr. Helen Fisher is a biological anthropologist who is a leading expert on the biology of love and attraction. I asked her what she thought of this #BadAdvice. "It's absolutely fallacious," she said. "It is based on absolutely nothing. I don't know of any data that shows it . . . and I've read a tremendous amount of data from around the world [regarding] all kinds of people who fall in love who have no understanding of Western psychology and have never heard the statement that you're supposed to love yourself before you love anybody else. It just does not work. It's not supported by brain circuitry." (So there.)

Fisher's research shows what the brain looks like when it's on love. Notice I'm not saying "in love." Know why? Because Fisher found that during the early phase of a relationship, a part of the brain called the ventral tegmental area, or VTA, tells certain cells to start pumping out dopamine—one of those powerful feel-good hormones. Another stimulus that triggers the same response is cocaine. But unlike cocaine, the high from Romantic Love is ongoing. Your mind isn't just taking a quick dip in those feel-good chemicals—it's marinating in them. Holy shit! Your brain just turned into the world's most generous drug dealer. Fisher believes this explains why Romantic Love can cause you to lose your sense of yourself. You become obsessed with the other person, almost as if addicted to them. If your brain is a drug dealer, the one you love is its supplier. The VTA is located in that deep, primal part of the brain associated with your basic survival instincts and cravings called the reptilian core. Fisher describes the VTA as "below your emotions." But your instinctive, biological ability to love doesn't stop inside you; it also connects you to the one you love.

Dr. Stephen Porges is a researcher and professor of psychiatry. His research has revealed that your body involuntarily responds to physical signals from the people you interact with. So when the person who sets your heart, brain, and body on fire feels the same about you, the tone of their voice, their facial expressions, and other subtle cues will reflect it. Your body responds by mellowing out to let you enjoy the moment and connect with this person: Your heart rate slows, your breath deepens, even your ears adjust so that you can listen better.

All of this happens without your decision or intention. The act of loving is involuntary, like breathing, eating, and sleeping. It is a hallmark of what makes you human. So not only are you born able to love, you're already doing it. In the throes of an amorous mania, we never really consider this biological inevitability. But you don't need to fully comprehend love before you can love, just as you don't need to understand how your lungs work before you can breathe. Because it's not the *if* of love you need to consider, but the *how*. After all, just because you're Italian doesn't mean you can cook spaghetti. (I speak from my own experience as an Italian who can't cook spaghetti.)

All of this science and data beg the question: If Romantic Love is such a biological inevitability, why do we all keep fucking it up? But what if you're *not* fucking up at love? What if you're already an expert, and perfectly imperfect at loving others? According to your own biochemistry, you are. The problem isn't that you don't know how to love; it's that you exist in a state of doubt and conflict with your own biology. #BadAdvice will almost always lead you to this conflicted state. And it has a sidekick to help out.

Advertising: The Art of Making You Forget You Already Have Everything You Need

Billions of dollars are spent every year to make you feel like shit, and those dollars are advertising dollars. You are always under a constant barrage of ads. Those ads may not all sell the same thing, but nearly all of them *say* the same thing: "You don't want to be a fat/ugly/boring/lonely bitch do you? Then buy this!" It's a pervasive and insidious meta-message that contributes to the mindfuck of *You Can't Love Anyone Until You Love Yourself*. How can you love yourself if you're twisted up in the cultural meta-message that you're somehow less-than, unworthy, or otherwise defective? If you're a woman, this message hits you extra hard.

From the time they are little girls onward, women are taught to feel shame over their bodies. Dove soap's "Choose Beautiful" campaign found that less than 4 percent of women in our society consider themselves beautiful. A report released in 2016 by the Australian organization Jean Hailes for Women's Health found that women were more afraid of being fat than getting cancer. A research brief from Common Sense Media found that the average girl goes on her first diet at age eight. And yet, on the other side of the world, the island nation of Fiji was immune to this kind of self-hate. "You've gained weight" was considered a compliment there . . . until Fiji began pumping in American TV shows and commercials. It took fewer than five years for adolescent girls' self-esteem to crater. Young Fijian women suddenly felt "too heavy" and were being fat-shamed by their peers.

So it's no coincidence that millions of women across the world manifest the same kind of self-loathing. We're conditioned to self-hate, yet expected to self-love. *You Can't Love Anyone Until You Love Your Fat, Ugly Self.*

They Keep Selling It Because We Keep Buying It

While you're being coerced into trying to buy away your self-hate, you're simultaneously told that loving yourself fixes everything. Do a Google image search for "love yourself" and you'll be buried for days in sappy stock photos of hearts, birds, flowers, solitary lighthouses, and other assorted soft-focus bullshit, all captioned with this #BadAdvice. It's also a bona fide money maker; we're branding this #BadAdvice: "Love yourself," purrs Justin Bieber. K-Pop boy band BTS created a musical soap opera called the "Love Yourself" series. And then there are those regular peeps who just "like" their own Facebook statuses.

But even if you *could* somehow love yourself first, you'd still keep that shit to yourself . . . unless you're Gucci Mane, tweeting "I Love Me" on the regs. Self-love wouldn't be something you'd list on your online profile. *About me: I love myself. DTF.* No one wants to hang out with a narcissistic asshole even if they are DTF (well, maybe just once for that initial F, but after that, you'd be DTF as in *Deciding to Forget*). It's hard to say "I love myself" and not sound like a conceited bastard. But "I hate myself" doesn't sound any better. Self-loathing is a shitty aphrodisiac.

The dark irony is that while self-love may be a self-help fantasy, self-hate is often all too real. And the impossibility of loving yourself doesn't change the fact that so much around you is still conditioning you toward self-hate. There is no doubt that self-hate is a negative attribute that pollutes the way you love others, and you might think self-love would be the obvious replacement for self-hate. But it isn't. *Because self-love is a myth.* And yet, here we are, millions of ass-backwards motherfuckers trying to follow the #BadAdvice to love ourselves *first*, while being conditioned to self-hate.

For all the pressure and expectation for you to *Love Yourself, Love Yourself, Love Yourself*, nobody offers you any idea of *how* to do it. You know why? I'll let Helen Fisher explain: "You can't love yourself. It's an emotion that evolved so that you can make a connection with somebody else." Loving other people is a biological inevitability. Loving yourself is a biological *impossibility*. But if the whole point of this chapter, let alone the whole point of this book, let alone the whole point of the entire fucking self-help genre, is to learn how to really love yourself, and that's impossible . . . *then what the fuck are we doing?* Science confirms that Romantic Love exists exclusively as an interactional process between people, not the internal process of an individual, aka "loving yourself." Which is why the antidote to self-hate doesn't spring from a daydream of self-love, but the reality of *self-care*.

Loving Someone Else Means Caring for Yourself

High school health class might teach you some shit about where you can expect to start growing hair, why drugs are bad, and how to use a condom, but nobody is really taught self-care for the heart and mind. If you're lucky, you might find a famous self-help guru to teach you. (But a lot of those TV shrinks are full of shit . . . *yeah, I know.*) Your biology ensures that you'll love people no matter what. But you will love *well* only when you know how to take care of your heart and mind.

And that means so much more than maintaining your cardio routine, being a good flosser, and knowing how to use a condom. (Not that those things aren't important: In fact, sometimes mastering the first two leads to needing to know how to do the third.) You need to know more. You need to be able to remind yourself of your own worth. You have to know how to set healthy limits for yourself. You need to know when it's time to tell yourself "no" and when to tell yourself "yes." You need to be confident that you can depend on yourself, and others need to feel confident they can depend on you. You need to know more than how to feed yourself healthy foods, you need to know how to feed your heart. What this adds up to is that *true self-care is the ability to parent yourself.* When you know you can parent yourself, you will know you can love well. That brings us to this chapter's #GoodAdvice:

You'll Love Like a Motherfucker When You Know How to Mutha Yourself #GOODADVICE

Let's get this out of the way up front: There's a reason this chapter's #GoodAdvice is to *Mutha Yourself* and not to *Mother Yourself.* Mothers are great. I'm one myself. But a mother is not a *Mutha.* I mean just look at the word *Mutha.* Say it with me: *Mmmmmuuuuuthaaaa.* Really bring the air up from your center, put some power in it, and say it again: *Mutha.* Make it sound like what it is: something strong and wise coming from deep within you. And. It's. BIG! According to the Urban Dictionary (the twenty-first century's answer to Webster's), *Mutha* is a word used to exaggerate an amount, e.g., *the Mutha load*. So if a casting call went out for someone to play the role of *Mutha*, who would you cast? Tami Roman? Ru Paul? Ruth Bader Ginsburg? Snoop Dogg? Who would your *Mutha* be?

Being able to *Mutha Yourself* isn't about your parents; *it's about learning to parent yourself.* Because no matter how great or how shitty your parents were, you're an adult now. It's on you to give yourself what your parents either did or didn't give you. And that's more than eating your veggies and making your bed. When you parent yourself, you create and cultivate your own source of inner comfort, nurturing, protection, and guidance. And *that* is what primes you to love well—not learning to love yourself first. Which is why I'm telling you to *Mutha Yourself.* Your own *Mutha* is already within you, waiting for your invitation to enter your life. It's an invitation you send through forgiveness.

With Forgiveness, the Heart Begins to Heal

Forgive yourself for everything you've done from birth up until now. And if there's something in your past that you're torturing yourself over, take comfort in this: *You* probably remember what you believe to be The Worst Thing You Ever Did more clearly than anyone else. They probably don't remember what you believe to be The Worst Thing You Ever Did. Or, if they do, they don't give a shit. Your inner *Mutha* definitely doesn't give a shit.

Even so, if you feel that reaching out to someone and offering them a personal apology is what *you* need to do to forgive yourself, then do that. Never forget that you have the ability to make things right. So forgive yourself. Say it out loud: "I forgive myself." Keep repeating it until you do. "Loving yourself" is impossible. Forgiving yourself is mandatory.

You've also suffered enough for whatever's been done *to* you. Forgive yourself for all that. You know what your inner *Mutha* would tell you? She'd tell you that you're not responsible for the horrible behavior of the cruel assholes of the world. Don't blame yourself for crossing their paths. Shame is a spiritual toxin. Someone else's shitty behavior is nothing for you to be ashamed of. And you better fucking believe that who *you* are is nothing to be ashamed of. The #BadAdvice of *You Can't Love Anyone Until You Love Yourself* will help you feel shame, because you haven't figured out how to "love yourself." Wanna get rid of shame? *Mutha Yourself.* Recognize your baseless shame for what it is: a poison. It pollutes your psyche, leads you to doubt your instincts, and encourages you to believe yourself unworthy of love.

Your *Mutha* knows better. Listen to her.

Don't Lean into Pain and Don't Let Pain Lean into You

When I was a kid, my mother beat the shit out of me. Because that's how overwhelmed, underprepared teen moms often rolled in 1972 (and some still do). But when my therapist asked me, "When did your mom love you?," my world changed. I realized all that pain and negativity coexisted with the love I felt for my mom *and the love she felt for me*. I was able to perceive the multiple truths of our relationship. My mom could love me very much *and* be a shitty parent. It didn't excuse the abuse, but it helped me see my mom as an imperfect human, not a villain.

Your inner *Mutha* will tell you the same holds true in any relationship. Nobody has to be a villain to fuck up and hurt you. This doesn't mean you should accept or remain in an unhealthy relationship, but casting the roles of victim and villain creates false limits in your heart and cements you in pain and negativity. Recognize the coexisting truths that someone can mean you no harm *and* still be a reckless asshole. You'll spend less time in pain the less you lean into it.

Also be aware that leaning into pain can become addictive in its own right. Simply *feeling* anything can sometimes help you feel alive, and we are sensation-seeking creatures. Spend too much time with the same pain, and it'll convince you it's not pain anymore. You don't want to become habituated to familiar dysfunction. *Mutha Yourself*, and *Stop Leaning into Pain.*

When you stop leaning into pain, *be sure not to let pain lean into you.* Sometimes the world can help you feel small and powerless. That's because you have to share it with bigots, bullies, and assholes. These are the people who try to tell you who you are, how to act, who you can love, what you can do, and who you can be—sometimes without ever knowing your name, hearing your voice, or seeing your face. They don't see you as you are because *they can't see you at all*. You're an involuntary symbol for something they need to be true.

Love and relationships aren't immune to this dynamic. Your uniqueness is an asset, not an obstacle to someone's plans to change, fix, or remake you in their own image. You aren't here to absorb and take the shape of someone else's pain. Do not accept abuse—ever. Stay away from abusive assholes. This includes the sadistic cowards of the internet who confuse anonymity with courage. They just don't have the guts to be assholes in real life.

Muthas are protectors. *Mutha Yourself* and Protect Yourself: Stay away from assholes. Don't allow them to lean into you, don't try to change them, don't try to save them. Walk away. It doesn't matter what happened, nobody earns an asshole license.

Don't Collect Red Flags: Take the First One as Your Cue to Move On

If you find yourself consistently mismatched in love (loving the "wrong" person), you might be in the habit of talking yourself out of what you already know—aka ignoring your instincts. Your inner *Mutha* can't text or call you, but she can still send you messages through your instincts. So when someone says or does something that waves a bright red flag in your face, don't ignore it. Your *Mutha*, aka your instincts, is talking to you.

Look, I know it's a real bummer to discover that the reality of who someone is doesn't match with the reality of who you wanted them to be, but don't start up a collection of ignored red flags. Don't excuse the truth because you'd rather believe what you know to be false. And look, I get it—you're the kind of person who sees the best in people. That's an admirable quality. Never lose that. But your inner *Mutha* knows the difference between seeing the best in someone and seeing what you *want* to see in someone. A red flag is a signal to *Mutha Yourself* and GTFO.

Have Faith in the Goodness of Humans, Especially You

Make a daily list of your undeniable good. Don't confuse this with staring into the mirror and parroting sappy self-help bullshit you don't believe. Your *Mutha* never bullshits you. Scientific data show it's not the truth of an affirmation but your belief in it that makes it effective. Research even shows that trying to self-affirm things you don't really believe can have harmful effects. So to hell with affirmations. Just as you shifted your perspective from self-love to self-care, turn away from the idea of affirmations and instead hone in on your verifiable attributes. It's your job to find real-world evidence for the things you do well and list them. *I am good at . . . I've learned how to . . . People depend on me for . . .* and so on.

Making a daily list both keeps your undeniable good in the front of your mind and primes you to reveal it to others. If you're having trouble with this, try to see yourself as those who love you do. When the shit hits the fan in my own life, at those times when I can think of *nothing* good about myself, I push myself to see me through the eyes of my husband, my parents, my kids, my friends. Their love and presence in my life give me the evidence I need when I doubt my own goodness. You can do the same with the ones you love. Because even when you can *Mutha Yourself* like a motherfucker, sometimes you need the jump-start of someone else's example.

Which leads me to my next point: Your inner *Mutha* keeps tabs on the crowd you run with. It's not that she's breathing down your neck, but she wants to remind you that *people are contagious*. What you consistently see in other people shapes what you see in yourself. When you spend your time with people who feed goodness into your life, you'll see that goodness reflected in yourself. And if you always hang out with creeps who ooze negativity, well, ask your inner *Mutha* and she'll tell you, "You can't soar with the eagles when you flock with the turkeys."

Take some time and consider the people you're closest to. Where is the good and who is it coming from? Stick with them. The people who bring the most good into your life bring out the most good in you. If you have trouble finding anyone matching this description, start looking for them. Ask your *Mutha* to set up a play date. (I kid. *Muthas* don't do play dates.)

If You're Constantly Checking Your Phone, Don't Forget to Check Your Head

Do you treat yourself as well as you treat your smartphone? Because I'm sure when that little battery icon turns red, the charger's hooked up faster than a freshman on spring break. When it's update time, I bet that shit is downloaded and installed before you finish your coffee. But do you do the same for yourself when *you* need a recharge? How do you know when your psyche's software needs an update? *How do you know when you need a break?* It's hard to know these things when everyone expects an instant response to everything. Well, everyone except your *Mutha*. She's hip: She knows when you've had too much screen time and need to unplug.

It's those moments when you're feeling overworked, overwhelmed, and out of time that you need to do less, not try to do more. Disconnect from whatever stress generators are present and just *be* in stillness, even if for just five minutes. And if it doesn't feel like you have five minutes . . . *tough! Figure out what YOU need to do to recharge.* Shit, you know what your f'n phone needs! It's your responsibility to know what *you* need. For example, I know that I need ten minutes to recover from a client session but two days to bounce back from the DMV. Your inner *Mutha* stands firm on this shit: *You take care of that goddamn phone better than you take care of yourself. Gimmie it! Now go outside.*

Seriously, every minute of your life is a piece of the *life-*

time you are living. That time belongs to you, and *only* you. You're allowed to slow things down: You decide the tempo of conversations, the making of decisions, the pace with which you respond to things—all of it. *Your life-time is yours to live.* And your inner *Mutha* knows that's just as true when you're feeling underwhelmed, uninspired, or just plain bored. *"You bored? You're smart, go find somethin' to do."* Leave your comfort zone. Try new things, learn new things, do new things. Seeking out new experiences creates a momentum of real growth and achievement. This is your one shot at life. Find adventure. Reclaim your time.

Don't Let the Wisdom of Childhood Evaporate with Age

You may take it for granted, but your adulthood is proof that you've already overcome whatever childhood struggles you had to face. Which means that you can tell yourself now what you needed to hear then. Your inner *Mutha* is really just the name we're giving to your innate strengths, wisdom, and abilities—you know, the things #BadAdvice wants you to deny. When that happens, you lose touch with that fiery, childlike element within.

To reconnect with that confident, creative, carefree spark in the present (aka your inner *Mutha*) Mutha Your Past Self. Ask yourself this question, and your *Mutha* will answer: *What are the two words you would tell your younger self?*

Whatever you think you'd tell your younger self, say it to yourself now. Write those two words down on a pocket-sized card, and always keep it with you. Like a note in your lunch-box, it's tangible proof and guidance from your *Mutha*. I've done this. My two words are, "Fear Nothing." Find the two words that carry your truth and repeat them to yourself over and over. You have boundless creativity and energy to tap into. Undim them now.

Take Good Care of Your Body:
No Returns or Exchanges

Your inner *Mutha* knows that all these handy-dandy self-care tips won't count for shit if you're not taking *physical* care of yourself. *"Huh? It's Saturday. It's gorgeous out. I don't care what you do, but you ain't sittin' in front of that fuck'n TV all day."* Find *some* kind of physical activity that you enjoy—or even hate; just make sure it's something you can commit to. Don't eat a ton of shit food. Don't do drugs. You're probably at least somewhat aware of this. But just to annoy you, here are more stats! Regular exercise strengthens bones, blood vessels, your immune system, and the rest of your body; it eases stress, helps prevent serious illnesses like diabetes and cancer, and makes you smarter (all the dumb gym rats you know notwithstanding). Oh yeah, you'll also get in shape. (Just remember, we're not all supposed to be the same shape.)

Your inner *Mutha* wants you to feel good, and to feel good

about your body. That includes orgasms. (See, this would be weird if it were your actual mother we were talking about, but since your inner *Mutha* is really you, we're all good.) The psychological and physical benefits that, ahem, *come* from orgasms are hard, scientific facts. Orgasms improve sleep and circulation, ease stress, prolong life, increase production of health-promoting hormones . . . and the list goes on.

There's no reason for you to miss out on any of this great stuff just because you're dolo for the time being. If no one's around to give you an orgasm, give one to yourself. Don't be afraid or ashamed of your body. Know where your clitoris is located and touch her, or explore around the head, underside, and frenulum of your penis. Set all your electronic devices to Do Not Disturb (well, *almost* all your devices) and take the time to discover what makes you feel good. As in *really* good. That's a discovery you'll be able to share with your partner(s) as well. Orgasms are good for you, you deserve to have as many as you want, and a self-help book from a major publisher is instructing you to masturbate for good health. You're welcome. I promise you, your inner *Mutha* agrees with me.

There's Nothing to Be Afraid of and Sex Is Good for You: Have a Nice Day

Who was the asshole who decided it wasn't proper to talk about sex? Our culture's fucked up view of love influences our fucked up view of sex. We get conflicting messages. On the one hand, you get the standard religion-rooted meta-message that sex is dirty and gross and bad . . . unless it's being used to sell you booze, a sports car, or a loofa, or whatever. But at the personal level, we attach all kinds of power games to sex. Like "Don't fuck 'til the third date." Your inner *Mutha* will call bullshit on that before you finish asking her the question. *My* inner *Mutha* was totally stoked when my husband and I fucked on the first date. Twenty years later, we're still fucking and she's still stoked. When everyone's a consenting adult, there's no reason to wait or feel weird or bad about fucking. And when you do fuck someone, be it for the first or thousandth time, you owe it to each other to *fuck well*. And your inner *Mutha* (*definitely* not your mother) will tell you to start by putting your honey where your mouth is. See Below.

No matter your gender or orientation, oral sex is one of life's greatest pleasures and responsibilities. You and your partner owe it to yourselves and each other to give and get it. The comedian Bill Maher once summed up the nature of oral sex in a relationship as "I'll do something that disgusts me if you do something that disgusts you" (Note: I'm paraphrasing). Not that giving head is disgusting to begin with, but you get the point: reciprocity. And while we're on the subject, don't be withholding from your partner or otherwise weaponize sex. Sex is a great way to smooth over the ruptures of an argument, but fighting shouldn't be a prerequisite for fucking. We all love make-up sex, but intimacy doesn't need conflict for an appetizer. *Mutha* your libido, and don't fetishize conflict.

Part of Caring for Those You Love
Is Caring for Yourself

When you *Mutha Yourself*, the long-term payoff is self-confidence. What does this have to do with you loving someone else? It has to do with YOU, because *you* are what you bring to the relationship. Genuine confidence is what enables you to reveal your best, both to yourself and to others. You don't have to worry about "loving yourself first" when you're already confident that you're worthy of loving and being loved. You are consciously maintaining and creating an undeniable source of self-confidence. And unlike a narcissistic illusion of self-love, self-confidence *is* one hell of an aphrodisiac.

Even if you haven't met that person already, someone (most likely *multiple* someones) is ready to fall in love with the unique, undeniable goodness that is you. I don't just mean there are people out there who would be stoked to fuck you. (Although those peeps are out there too.) I'm talking about real, deep, good-kind-of-crazy-making Romantic Love. Helen Fisher theorizes that you have a Romantic Love drive, separate from your sex drive. Because while your sex drive tells you to get out there and fuck as many different mates as possible, your Romantic Love drive wants you to, as Fisher puts it, "conserve your mating energy" for one specific individual: an ideal mate. According to the theory, an ideal mate will result in ideal offspring . . . following some ideal sex, of course. Romantic Love is more than a possibility for you, *it's inevitable*.

Maybe you're in love right now, or about to be. Anyone can and will fall in love. But only those who can *Mutha Themselves* will know how to love and be loved *well*.

We're on This Planet to Love Each Other; Everything Else Is a Distraction

Now that you can *Mutha Yourself*, imagine yourself and that proverbial Special Someone at the magic moment of a mutual Swipe Right. After forty-eight hours of sexting and one phone call, you meet in a public place. If you pass each other's Creep Tests (*Mutha* Approved!), you friend each other on all relevant social media outlets and maybe take the Big Step and (gasp!) *change the relationship status in your profile*. Your brain is soaking in dopamine and other feel-good hormones, driving you temporarily insane. Congratulations, you're both *on* love. But this probably isn't your first ride on the love roller-coaster. You've been burned. You've been fucked over. You've been hurt. Love does not give a shit about any of that—you're strapped in on a ride that's been running for as long as humans have been loving. Shit's about to go crazy. Literally so.

The ancient philosopher Plato defined love as ". . . a serious mental disease." Spanish poet Pedro Calderón de la Barca said that "When love is not madness, it is not love." Or as Madonna so famously confessed, "I've never wanted anyone like this, it's all brand new . . . I'm crazy for you." It's true. Love really does make us go crazy. And let's be honest here: romantic turmoil sucks. What else could drive a grown-ass adult to lie sobbing, facedown on the bathroom floor with tears and snot soaking into the rug? (Shared with the permission of a client.)

Once you've been there, *you know*. And at some point you will ask yourself, *Was this my fault?* Ask your inner *Mutha* and she'll tell you, *It's not your fault. It's love. Sometimes shit happens and no one's to blame.* But you won't hear your inner *Mutha* if you're listening to #BadAdvice. Ask the #BadAdvice of *You Can't Love Anyone Until You Love Yourself* whether you're to blame, here's the answer you'll get: *It* was *your fault. You loved the wrong person.* Or: *You loved the right person the wrong way. It's your fault because you don't know how to love. It's your fault because you don't love yourself. You Can't Love Anyone Until You Love Yourself.*

Love is a certified mania-maker, a notorious heart-breaker, and even sometimes an earth-shaker, but it isn't a memory-eraser. Even when you're steeping in dopamine from new love, you haven't forgotten that time Love left you crying on the bathroom floor. *You're afraid.* You shift into Fight, Flight, or Freeze when what you really want to do is Fantasize, French Kiss, or Fuck. Unlike love, you *can* choose whether or not you submit to fear. Don't expect any #BadAdvice to clear away your fear: For that, go ask your *Mutha*.

There Can Be No Love Without Courage

It's 2:32 p.m. on a Tuesday, and you are freaking the fuck out because you haven't texted with your sweetie in the past twenty-six minutes. Or maybe it's been two loooooong days since you've seen each other. Do you text? Do you call? *I'm not loving myself first. That's why I'm already fucking things up again, just like I always do.* Maybe you go to the gym more, meditate, or do whatever else to try to somehow love yourself. And maybe in some secret, superstitious corner of your being, you want to believe that being busy and away from your phone will make the text or call come in. Because there's no way in hell you want to look desperate or vulnerable. Otherwise, this person you love might think that you (gasp!) want to talk to them.

All of those futile variations of trying to "love yourself first" are based in fear, the fear of rejection. But you're afraid of being rejected by the same person you want to get closer to. You can't attempt to avoid risking rejection and try to get closer to someone at the same time. Hence all the stupid "love games" we play: waiting to call someone after a great date, expecting partners to read minds, or holding back on sharing what you really feel.

This is the illusion we mistake for love in the age of instant Tinder/Grindr gratification. They're all signs of an effort to avoid potential rejection, but you're simultaneously avoiding potential connection: One can't exist without the other. In trying to cope with the possibility of pain that will forever be inseparable from the joy of love, we've deceived ourselves into believing that the person who cares less wins. But I'm here to tell you: The person who cares less, gets less.

So how do you *Mutha Yourself* through the intersection

of love and fear? You don't stand there staring at the green light wondering whether it's *really* green—*you fucking go.* Because even if you forget, your inner *Mutha* always remembers that your life-time is far too precious to waste on bullshit. And these games are *always* bullshit. Text first. Call first. Don't force yourself to wait on replying. Share what you feel in the moment you feel it. Say "I love you" first. The games end when you decide you're not playing. When there are no games, there are no rules. The limits that you thought existed on love and on you at last appear as the illusions they are, before finally disappearing. *You Can't Love Anyone Until You Love Yourself* is the first to vanish, because you know that the love you feel is real. It's so real, in fact, that it reached in and physically activated the deepest part of your being. Listen to your Inner *Mutha*: *Be courageous in love.*

Parents don't want their kids to get hurt, which is why they tell younger ones to watch for traffic in the street and older ones to watch their backs in love. A lot of people hang on to both of those habits. So the advice you get from your *Mutha* can feel counterintuitive: *Lean into love. The love you feel is yours, even when it's not reciprocated.* Reciprocation isn't love, it's acceptance. The feeling of acceptance is part of love, but not all of it. Or as the character Donald in Charlie Kaufman's *Adaptation* said: "I loved Sarah, Charles. It was mine, that love. I owned it. Even Sarah didn't have the right to take it away. I can love whoever I want. . . . You are what you love, not what loves you." The love you keep within your heart is uniquely and solely yours. Lean into love, and lean in deep.

Here's the thing: Nothing great happens without risk and vulnerability. Love can thrive between you and someone else only when you allow yourself to be vulnerable. It takes time for a relationship to ripen enough to sustain vulnerability. But you've got an oxytocin mushroom cloud rising over your brain. Who has time to wait for vulnerability? And there's more chemical craze coming. All those shared moments of joy, laughter, and intimacy trigger releases of oxytocin, often called the "love hormone." You will feel even more connected to your partner because, not just emotionally but *chemically*, you are. But that connection needs time to strengthen so it can support real trust; otherwise, it can overload and short out.

Trying to *Love Yourself First* can't help you be vulnerable. Trying to follow that #BadAdvice makes you the opposite of vulnerable. But when you *Mutha Yourself*, you'll have the confidence and clarity to know how and when to let yourself be vulnerable. You'll understand that vulnerability on a first date could be as simple as saying, "I had a really great time tonight; I'd love to go out again." You're sharing genuine emotions that might not be returned, and you're opening the door to the unknown. Your date could give you a blank look and say, "Meh." But that person could also say, "Me too!" Vulnerability is like muscle memory in a relationship. When you make the effort to sustain it over time, you gradually achieve the state of what Zen philosophy describes as "effortless effort."

Oversharing Isn't Being Vulnerable

Ever been on a date, or just meeting someone new for the first time, and from out of nowhere they're sharing an unbelievably intimate piece of information about themselves or their past? Now you've got a side of WTF covered in awkward sauce to go with your dinner. That's *oversharing*. A lot of the time, oversharing is just a failed attempt to manage shame. If you're scared that someone will discover something you're ashamed of, oversharing can seem like a way to take control and beat them to it. Maybe this is something you do. Sometimes shame has nothing to do with it. You might be oversharing because you don't trust yourself to allow the nature of the relationship to unfold organically. But instead of bringing you closer together, oversharing pushes people away from you. It's trotting out your personal horror show to avoid being vulnerable.

So how can you tell when you're edging closer to oversharing? Check in with your inner *Mutha*. *"Can I trust this person with this information?"* Then she'll do the classic wise-advice thingy and answer your question with a question. *"Well, have they earned the right to be trusted that much? Have they had time to prove themselves worthy of your story, your intimacy, your vulnerability?"* Those are all things you build together, and they're gradually measured out through timing and dosage. Vulnerability isn't throwing your secrets at someone: It's letting someone know the secret you in a deliberate way, and that happens over time. Which is why there are times when being able to *Mutha Yourself* simply means knowing when to shut up.

Nobody Likes a Cruise on the
USS *Judgmental*: Bring That Ship Back to Port

When the one you love confides in you, responding with empathy and compassion sends the message that that person matters to you. If you want to make them feel loved, you sure as shit won't try to *Love Yourself First*. So don't get judgy when someone's reality doesn't conform to yours. Harsh judgment invalidates your partner and makes you look like an insensitive jackass. Nobody feels loved when someone judges them. *Mutha Yourself* and know the difference between keeping your side of the street clean and just being a judgy asshole.

But don't be so afraid of being judgmental that you stop using good judgment. Because when you *Mutha Yourself,* you don't confuse the two. You're not being judgmental when you decide to take your partner's car keys if they've had too much to drink. That's exercising good judgment (and probably saving lives). Being judgmental is thinking you're a better person because you didn't make the same mistake.

Love: A Fragile yet Indestructible
Constant of the Human Condition

You Can't Love Anyone Until You Love Yourself makes as much sense as telling someone *You Can't Eat Anything Until You Eat Yourself* (no matter what context you put the word "eat" in). Loving and eating are instinctive biological functions; you're born knowing how to do them. But what makes this #BadAdvice so seductive is its promise that you can love without risking pain. That flawed logic will stab you in the back. Going by this #BadAdvice, it's your fault when your heart gets broken: You loved the wrong person, because you don't know how to love. And you don't know how to love because *you didn't learn to love yourself first.* A part of you immediately senses that this #BadAdvice is bullshit: your inner *Mutha.* She recognizes *You Can't Love Anyone Until You Love Yourself* for the destructive bullshit it is. And because your inner *Mutha* is such a badass, I'll let her close out this chapter:

The question isn't whether you're going to love anyone. The question is how. How will you love? Will you love with fear, or will you love courageously? Will you love in vulnerability, or will you love in shame? Will you love in doubt, or will you love with confidence? Are you gonna try to love yourself first? 'Cause that shit ain't gonna work. Step up, listen to me, and Mutha Yourself.

YOU'LL LOVE LIKE A MOTHERFUCKER WHEN
YOU KNOW HOW TO MUTHA YOURSELF
#GOODADVICE

3

EXPECTATIONS LEAD TO
DISAPPOINTMENT

Expectations Lead to Disappointment. Isn't that a cheery no-
tion to hang your hat on? But why half-ass it and stop with
expectations? Why not whole-ass it and look at everything
in your life in that way: *Sleeping Leads to Nightmares. Dating Leads to Dumping. Puppies Lead to Dead Dogs. Expectations Lead to Disappointment* is #BadAdvice because, among
other reasons, it's self-contradictory. The belief that none of
your expectations can ever be met *is itself an expectation.*
It's a sucker-punch of pessimism that offers you *zero* guidance. *Expectations Lead to Disappointment* is a statement
without imperative, like *Life Sucks and Then You Die.* And
don't try to tell me that this shit is #RealTalk, or that pushing this psychological snake oil on yourself or anyone else
is proof of your street-cred—as if giving up on finding any

kind of satisfaction in life is a sign of worldly sophistication instead of emotional cowardice. Expectation and disappointment are emotions. They're unavoidable. Which is why this #BadAdvice qualifies for #BullshitAdvice.

We've been following this #BadAdvice for centuries. "Blessed is the man who expects nothing, for he shall never be disappointed," mused the English poet Alexander Pope. "Oft expectation fails, and most oft there where most it promises," wrote Mr. Shakespeare. "If you expect nothing from somebody you are never disappointed," said Sylvia Plath in *The Bell Jar*. According to Ayn Rand, freedom means, "To ask nothing. To expect nothing. To depend on nothing." (Although Ayn may have confused "freedom" with "prison.") And don't forget that Negative Nancy who tweeted "Expectations lead to disappointment" just last week.

For as long as we've been bullshitting ourselves, this #BadAdvice never gets any truer. But what makes this #BadAdvice such a sticky idea is how badly people want it to be true. Who wouldn't want a master control switch on their feelings? If you had a choice to opt out on disappointment, wouldn't you take it? Shit, sometimes *I* wouldn't mind it being true. *Disappointment sucks*. But following this #BadAdvice is like trying to avoid food poisoning by avoiding food. If you expect to go through life without feeling disappointed, well, you're going to be disappointed because that expectation isn't going to be met. Disappointment is an inevitability of the human condition, because it's directly connected to another human inevitability: expectations.

It's an Unrealistic Expectation to Expect Someone to Give Up All Their Expectations

We need expectations to function. They're the building blocks of human society. You expect the airline pilot to know how to fly the plane and not be shitfaced in the cockpit. You expect not to find cockroaches in your salad. You expect to be closed up after surgery. Only an asshole would tell you *Expectations Lead to Disappointment* if any of those expectations went unmet.

Zoom out for a second, beyond you. The world is connected and powered by humanity's collective expectations. Not only are global markets a collection of expectations, they're expected to *beat* those expectations. Peace treaties between countries express their mutual expectation not to blow the shit out of each other. Every human on the earth goes to bed expecting the sun to rise in the morning. Those are more than just reasonable expectations; those are *necessary* expectations for civilization to keep going.

Your personal expectations are just as necessary to keep *you* going. Yes, they're that important. Maybe I don't know the exact details of your unique, personal expectations, but I can tell you right now, they're probably not out of control or unreasonable. How do I know? Look past the personal details, and what you find are universal *human* expectations. You expect to feel loved. You expect to feel heard. You expect to feel like you matter. Those are expectations worth having, *and worth feel-*

ing disappointed over. From your own personal expectations to those that sustain civilization, *Expectations Lead to Disappointment* denies the benefit and the need of expectations. *Expectations Lead to Disappointment* is worse than just #BadAdvice. It's even worse than #BullshitAdvice. It's #AntiHuman.

Expectation Is a Coming Attraction for Fulfillment

Your expectations are important. They're so important that evolution created a biochemical insurance policy to make sure you have them. Expectation cues a small dopamine release in your brain. Yes, *that* dopamine, the same feel-good chemical that soaks your brain when you're in love. If your expectation is met, your brain squirts out a little more dopamine. Your brain treats you to an even bigger hit if you get more than you were expecting. Like when you win the lottery *and* have your first three-way before 2 p.m. on a Saturday. But guess what? Just crossing the street sooner than you expected is enough for your brain to give you the juice.

Eating. Avoiding Pain. Screwing. Expectation. They're All Instincts, and They All Feel Good

Evolution's logic is simple: *Expectations are necessary to survival; therefore, make them feel good.* Making an action feel good is evolution's way of making sure you do it. It's part of what has given our species a survival edge. Which is why *ex-*

pecting to get what you want or need feels good. But evolution never does anything just because it feels good (possible exception: the clitoris). Usually, there's a utilitarian reason for it. Which is why if you told prehistoric humans that *Expectations Lead to Disappointment*, they'd boot you out of the cave.

I spoke to Harvard psychologist and expert on expectations Dr. Robert Rosenthal, and he commented: "If you've been out on the Serengeti with your friends and you discover there's one fewer friend because one was eaten by a tiger or lion, you come to associate tigers or lions with [the expectation of] being eaten. So there's a very strong survival advantage to knowing who likes to eat people." Expectations Lead to Not Being Tiger Shit.

Your Mind, Your Body, and Your World Move on a Current of Expectations

Your expectations are powerful. Beyond your brain chemistry, your expectations can influence your reality. In one study, researchers told people they were drinking better wine than they actually were. This expectation was enough to activate their brains' reward center to respond as if they were drinking Château Lafite Rothschild instead of Mad Dog 20/20.

And expectations can do more than save you money at the liquor store. Dr. Alberto Espay, a leading researcher in the treatment of Parkinson's disease, found that the symptoms of people with Parkinson's improved when they believed they'd been given an expensive drug. The miracle drug they responded so strongly to? Saline, aka salt water. Now look, I'm sure you already know about the placebo effect. But what's the psychological process behind it? Expectation. Espay's patients *expected* those results from the saline he gave them. A placebo tricks you into meeting your own expectations.

I was able to talk to Dr. Espay about his work, and his take on expectations blew me away. Espay wonders if it might be possible for doctors to prescribe expectations to help patients get better. "What if we *were* to make promises?," he asked. "What if we told patients, 'Here's a medication. . . . Based on everything I know about you, you should respond to this . . . and respond very well.'" Espay's not an outlier. Study after study and trial after trial reveal the power of the placebo effect, and the expectations behind it.

I'm not suggesting that happy thoughts can cure leprosy, but dismissing the value of your expectations is like Superman choosing to fly coach. The writer Alan Moore said that "the ultimate act of magic is to create something from nothing." It's possible your expectations exist at a very real intersection between science, magic, dreams, and reality. Expectations do more than just serve as a projection of what you want from the future. They can actually shape your future. In the words of journalist and author Kathryn Schulz, "The miracle of your mind isn't that you can see the world as it is. It's that you can see the world as it isn't."

So if expectations are so great, why do they get such a bad rap? Because they're not always met. And when an expectation isn't met, your brain does more than hold back on that next shot of dopamine: *Your existing dopamine levels take a nosedive.* The sudden drop in dopamine equals a sudden drop in emotions: You feel disappointed. That feeling sucks. Sometimes it sucks so bad, it hurts. Like, really hurts. So you promise yourself you'll never be disappointed again by never having expectations. That's a promise you'll never be able to keep, and an expectation that will never be met.

But here's the thing: Just like your expectations, disappointment is an involuntary biological process. Although it's painful and shitty, it does serve a purpose. Because sometimes you don't even realize an expectation exists *until* it goes unmet. The disappointment you feel in that moment is not just a sign of an unmet expectation; it's an alarm that you're not getting what you need.

The Pain of Disappointment Is the Distress Signal of an Unmet Need

Your emotions are messengers that carry information about you, and disappointment is no exception. The #BadAdvice of *Expectations Lead to Disappointment* stops disappointment from delivering an important message: *Find another way to get what you need, because whatever you're doing now isn't working.* Disappointment is an example of what behavioral psychologist B. F. Skinner termed "negative reinforcement." A lot of people confuse negative reinforcement with punishment, but that's not always the case. You experience negative reinforcement whenever you realize that taking a certain action removes something unpleasant from your life. For instance, you might decide to stop going on weeknight benders to remove the unpleasant experience of barfing in the copy room because you're hung over at work.

The involuntary emotional response of disappointment ensures that having an unmet expectation is a negative experience. Disappointment is evolution's way of kicking you in the ass to make sure you meet your needs, because an unmet expectation equals an unmet need. When you find a way to meet that unmet expectation and need, you help remove that feeling of disappointment. *Disappointment is an emotional cue saying that you need to adapt.* Following this #BadAdvice means ignoring one of your greatest human superpowers: your ability to adapt to meet your needs in the face of the unexpected. This includes everything from your most basic physical needs, to your needs to feel loved and safe, to your needs to find meaning, fulfillment, and joy. Expectations and disappointment both connect directly to your *Greatest Potential Self.* Which, through an unbelievably fortunate coincidence abbreviates as GPS, and makes for some damn #GoodAdvice.

Expectations Lead to Your GPS:
Greatest Potential Self #GOODADVICE

Unless you're Amish, you've probably used a GPS device to direct you from one spot to another. (If you are Amish and reading this, then you must be on your *Rumspringa*. Good luck, and make the choice that feels right for you!) Every one of your expectations directs you toward an emotion you want to feel, not a situation you want to be in. The #BadAdvice of *Expectations Lead to Disappointment* misleads you to believe that your expectations are only connected to a certain external outcome or situation, instead of the satisfaction of an inner need. For example, you might have an expectation that your best friend will keep you looped in on his or her birthday plans. This expectation doesn't spring from your burning desire to go to Benihana. It comes from your need to feel included by someone you care about, to feel like you matter to that person. That expectation *should* be met, because you deserve to feel loved, to feel important, to feel like you matter. You deserve all that and more because *those are basic human needs*. Fulfilling those needs keeps you cruising down life's road on a full tank. And in finding your own satisfaction and fulfillment, you help the people you're connected with to do the same. Like the way you helped your friend feel loved and needed by being at that Benihana birthday dinner. *That* is your Greatest Potential Self. When your expectations aren't met, your GPS speaks to you through your disappointment. Staying connected with your expectations *and* your disappointment keeps you tuned in to your internal GPS. And your GPS guides you toward the satisfaction of your needs. Your Greatest Potential Self is your built-in survival guide: Watch out for anyone who argues against it.

No matter how unfamiliar you might be with your own

expectations, I'm willing to bet you'd recognize the Voice of Expectation in a heartbeat. The Voice of Expectation is Karen Jacobsen—the steady voice of reason coming from your car's GPS, calmly telling you to "turn right" when you're about to lose your shit in traffic. So why is this GPS Lady also the Voice of Expectation? Because the GPS in your heart isn't that different from the GPS in your car. Both maintain a simultaneous awareness of where you are, where you want to be, and multiple ways to get there. Expectation and disappointment are irreplaceable guides to understanding your needs and how to meet them. Both give you an idea of where you are and where you want to go. Your Greatest Potential Self depends on them to help set your destination. Disappointment is nothing to be afraid of, so in the words of the GPS Lady . . . *Let's go!*

Don't Be Afraid to Ask for What You Want, Especially from Yourself

You can't get the most out of your GPS without having some idea of where you want to go. If you're unsure which needs and emotions your Greatest Potential Self is guiding you toward, then explore your expectations. Your expectations clue you in on what you want and where you want to go with your life. Exploring them helps you recognize the needs and emotions attached to your expectations. This enables you to become *conscious* of what you expect from yourself. When you're aware of the unmet need connected to that expectation, you're able to consider other potential ways to meet that need.

For example, have you ever found yourself caught up in the idea that what you do for a living defines you? As if your sole purpose and meaning in life is climbing that professional ladder. But no matter what your job is, it can't singularly fulfill your need for meaning, achievement, and purpose in life. Which is why if you expect it to, you'll wind up feeling disappointed. So maybe you get that promotion you've been working toward, and maybe you *do* feel happy . . . for like three days. But all too soon that gnawing, empty feeling of an unmet need creeps back in, and with it, disappointment. You feel disappointed because this thing that you worked so hard to achieve failed to fulfill you. And if you *didn't* get the promotion, this example still applies because you're still feeling disappointed on the other side of your expectations.

This is why it's vital to *question your disappointment.* Exploring your disappointment and everything connected to it enables you to recognize the unmet need at the root of your unmet expectations. When you know what need is unmet, you can start figuring out other ways to meet that need. Without questioning your disappointment, you're gonna have an even harder time piecing together how to satisfy the unmet need at the root of your disappointment.

It took me two master's degrees and a PhD to learn this. My diploma would come in the mail (I don't do graduations: Why make the people I love sit through three hours of names?), I'd open it up, look at it, and think to myself, *Am I enough now?* And the answer was always "no": I was looking for validation and approval on a piece of paper. It would be a few more years before I began to realize that it's my connections to everything and everyone in my life that make me enough, not a myopic focus on one corner of it. It's unrealistic to expect professional success or achievement to completely fulfill you. You might as well expect food to materialize in an empty fridge after you close and open the door.

So, get curious and ask yourself about everything you expect and everything you need from life. *What do I want? What do I need? What do I expect from myself? What do I expect from others? What do I expect from love? What do I expect from work? What do I expect from life?* Then go deeper and ask, *How do I expect to feel when my expectations are met?* The emotion you expect to feel points to the need your expectation expresses. So as you arrive at each of your answers, challenge it by asking yourself, *Is it realistic and reasonable for me to expect this?* If the answer is "no," then you need to adapt that expectation. But how do you know whether you're being unrealistic or not?

There's Absolutely No Room for Absolutes in a Life as Complex as Yours

Unrealistic expectations are easy to spot because they're almost always absolute. Absolute expectations give themselves away because they usually have words like "never" or "always" in them. *I should always be happy . . . I'm never gonna do what I want to . . . I always need to be right . . . My partner should always . . . My mother should always . . .* and so on. Absolute expectations leave no room for bending with reality and no room for your or anyone else's human fallibility. Inflexible expectations still express a valid emotional need, but they reflect a misguided belief that you can meet that emotional need in only one way.

Your Greatest Potential Self is GREAT, but it's also flawed and messy. You will fuck up, others will fuck up, expectations will go unmet, you will feel disappointed. But the more inflexible your expectations are, the more disappointment is gonna hurt. Inflexible expectations make disappointment feel like being stuck on a dead-end street in a world of only dead end streets. Your Greatest Potential Self sees disappointment for what it is: an obstacle to navigate around. The GPS Lady knows this too. It's why she sounds so confident and cheery when she pipes up and says "Recalculating route."

Your Greatest Potential Self Is Your Most Vulnerable Self

Your Greatest Potential Self uses both your expectations of others and their expectations of you as a guide. How? We are social animals who are designed to help each other feel things. And some things you can feel *only* when someone else helps you. You help make that happen through the connection of your interpersonal expectations.

One place you can see this most clearly in life is in the expectations of your romantic relationships. What you need from a relationship makes itself known through your expectations of your partner. Now, I realize that you might be inclined to freak the fuck out if some hypothetical early-stage-of-the-relationship-bae were to say to you, "Here's what I expect from our relationship." You'd probably take it as your cue to Unfriend, Block, and Flag as Inappropriate. But effectively communicating your expectations of someone actually sends a message of trust and vulnerability. *This is what I want to feel, and you are the only person I want to make me feel it.*

For example, you might realize that you expect a text from your partner every day because it helps you feel like you matter to them, and it could also help satisfy your need for consistency. After more than twenty years together, I *still* get jazzed when my husband sends me a good morning and a goodnight text. The comfort of consistency and feeling like you matter never get old. Just remember, it's not really the *text* that matters—*it's the way the text makes you feel.* So take the initiative: *You* be the one to start sending texts every morning and every night. Or better yet, call your partner (gasp!). Help your partner feel the love and dedication you want them to help you feel. You'll create a connection between both of your Greatest Potential Selves, and help each other get what you both need.

Let me give you an example from the Dr. V Archives. With five kids and two perpetually exhausted parents, my family didn't make a big deal out of birthdays when I was growing up. So I never saw my birthday, or anyone else's, as a big deal. Which is why it wasn't until a few years into our marriage that I started meeting my husband Matthew's expectation to remember his birthday. (I know! I'm such a jackass.) That happened only because every year he would forge my signature on a birthday card, mail it to himself, and jokingly thank me for it. But Matthew's expectations didn't feel aggressive. His humor helped me see his expectations as a reflection of his need to feel loved and acknowledged. Those goofy self-addressed birthday cards created connection between our Greatest Potential Selves. I found myself standing at that place where expectations intersect with science, magic, dreams, and reality. Understanding Matthew's expectations of me changed my self-expectations. It changed what I believe. It changed *me*. I make a big deal out of birthdays now. I send gift baskets to relatives I haven't seen in years—because people in general should celebrate each other more, especially on the day that marks the entry into the world of someone you love. (Matthew, consider this my formal apology.)

Why do these little things always seem to end up meaning so much? Because the daily text, the morning phone call, the birthday card, and whatever else send this message to the receiver: *You matter to me.* Making someone feel like they matter provides for one of their most basic emotional needs. Which is why communicating your expectations to your partner helps you both connect to your Greatest Potential Selves.

Expectations don't always lead to disappointment. They lead to love. They lead to connection. They lead to change. Expectations are avenues for us to inspire and change each other. More than just leading to your Greatest Potential Self, expectations bring you closer to the Greatest Potential Selves of the ones you love.

Our Greatest Potential Selves Connect in a Web of Expectations

A relationship doesn't have to be romantic to impact your GPS. A good friend might notice that you put yourself down all the time and share that with you, because they know you don't deserve it. *They* see your Greatest Potential Self at times when you don't. When a friend helps you calibrate your GPS, they help shift your self-expectations in a more positive direction. And if you realize that someone consistently shifts your self-expectations in a more *negative* direction, here's a hot tip: *That person is probably a shitty friend.*

And by the way, the influence between friendships and expectations flows both ways. For as much as your relationships can define and influence your expectations, your expectations also mold and shift your relationships.

Some of the people you learn the most from in life have no idea they're teaching you. You probably don't expect to be able to let your guard down with your co-workers in the same way as with your weekend party crew. And you most likely don't expect to find the same closeness, intimacy, and trust with the party crew as you do in your deeper, lasting friendships. When you recognize how your mutual expectations with other people define the boundaries of your relationships, you're also able to recognize when your expectations might be misconnected or misdirected.

Recognizing the limits of how deep your connection and trust with someone goes is an early lesson to learn. You wouldn't expect to head east by merging into the westbound lane, and friendships are no different. My friend asked someone she already knew was an irresponsible fuckup to housesit for her. When my friend got home, she discovered that the fuckup had eaten all the ice cream (Talenti) and stolen four months' worth of laundry quarters. You gotta go to the bank for that shit! Nobody's got laundry quarters just sitting around! "Should I be mad?" she asked me. My reply? "You feel how you feel, but you did entrust your home to a known irresponsible fuckup." Don't dive into a shallow relationship with deep expectations.

Expectations Are Involuntary, Meeting Them Is a Decision

Someone else's expectation of you is an expression of how that person wants *you* to help them meet a need and feel a certain way. Since you were little, your inner GPS has been shaped by the expectations of your family, friends, teachers, and others. But as a grown-ass adult, you have something you didn't have as a kid: autonomy. So how can you know whether someone's expectation of you is realistic and reasonable? Answer this question for yourself: *Is the help they're asking for reasonable, or are they asking you to do their emotional heavy lifting?* Your partner expecting you to help them feel loved by remembering their birthday is totally reasonable. Your partner expecting you to maintain a certain BMI because they've made you a narcissistic extension of their own body dysmorphic bullshit isn't. It's okay to disappoint someone when the only alternative is hurting yourself.

Along with your expectations and the expectations of other people, your Greatest Potential Self maintains expectations of the society you live in. These usually fall into the category of expectations that go unnoticed unless they're unmet: You expect the power company to keep the lights on. You expect your email to work. You expect new clips on your favorite porn site to appear semi-regularly. Then there are the expectations society places on you. Unless you're an asshole, you're probably unaware of meeting these expectations: *Don't text after the movie starts. Chew with your mouth closed. Don't rob banks.*

But then there are those *other* social expectations. The social expectations for you to be less than your Greatest Potential Self. They're usually based on things like your gender, age, profession, social status, or sexual orientation. And by definition they conflict with your GPS, because they expect you be less than who you really are. Those expectations need to be fucking challenged. Never forget that "normal" is the brand of insanity accepted by the most people. Challenging expectations puts you in good company. The people who make the biggest impact on the world are those with the courage to challenge oppressive social expectations: Mahatma Gandhi. Rosa Parks. Martin Luther King Jr. Malala Yousafzai. Cesar Chavez. Nelson Mandela. Harriet Tubman. Their courage helped them to face so much more than the pain of disappointment. They inspired others and gave humanity a glimpse of its Greatest Potential Self. The same potential and strength are in you. They originate from the same place as your expectations: your Greatest Potential Self. But your expectations aren't the only guidance your inner GPS has to offer. Because believe it or not, disappointment also directs you toward fulfillment.

You Are a Direct Descendant of Someone Who Survived the Ice Age; You Can Handle Disappointment

What's your go-to emotional position for disappointment? I'm an easy target for me to hit, so I usually default to blaming myself. I fall into negative thinking loops like *I'm not good enough, I should've known better, It's my fault*, etc. But I know other people who blame everyone except themselves: *People always fuck me over, They set me up to fail, Everyone else has it easy*, and so on. The emotional flood of disappointment can make you feel cut off from your GPS, so you need to reconnect. You do that in the same way you connected with your GPS to begin with—through curiosity. When you need to drive somewhere you've never been before, you search for the place with your GPS and go there. You can do the same with your inner GPS and search yourself. Explore your destructive, false narratives, because reality-testing defuses them.

For instance, you might feel like an unfuckable loser and doomed to die alone because your crush just turned you down. *Challenge that.* I mean, of course you're allowed to feel bad, because rejection (a breed of disappointment) blows. But do you *really* believe that out of the billions of people on Earth, this one person was your best, last hope to ever find love? Or do you think it just *might* be possible that you could find someone else? Activate your Greatest Potential Self and override the blame circuit. When you do this, you make room to replace negativity and undeserved shame with self-forgiveness.

If you need a kick start on forgiveness right now, remember this: *You're not wrong for having expectations; you're not wrong for feeling disappointed: You're human.* Your GPS depends on your expectations *and* your disappointments to help reroute you and guide you toward fulfillment and satisfaction. Do you really want to cut yourself off from that information? And remember: *This is disappointment, not death.* The trip's not over; you just need to recalculate your route. Your own curiosity about your expectations and disappointments can help you reconnect with your Greatest Potential Self.

For as unwanted and painful as it is, disappointment empowers you with the knowledge of how to satisfy your unmet needs and expectations. So if you're suffering through a deep disappointment now, know this: What you're feeling isn't a sign of failure; *it's evidence of courage*. It's evidence that you had the courage to try. You had the courage to love. You had the courage to make yourself heard. And courage is never wrong. You can never waste it, because you create it for yourself in infinite amounts. Your courage originates from the same thing that guides your expectations and supports you in disappointment: your Greatest Potential Self.

Don't Confuse "Never" with "Not Yet"

Disappointment is a kind of grief, which is why it can hurt so badly. It's a unique kind of grief, because you're mourning the loss of something you never had: a hoped-for future that will never happen. That doesn't mean you'll *never* get what you want or need. The answer isn't "no"; for now it's just "not yet." So step back and consider something. *What exactly in that future are you grieving for?* The granular details and mechanics of how that happens might differ from what you previously expected, but you *will* find another way to meet your needs. Your inner GPS will recalculate and point you in a new direction, and your inner GPS Lady will say *Let's go!* You'll no longer feel stuck in disappointment because you've begun moving through it. And even though it's great that you've got your engine running and you're starting to drive through disappointment, it doesn't mean you won't still feel disappointment. Yes, it's important to recognize and mourn whatever has been *really* lost, but it's equally important not to mistake "not yet" for "never."

The next time you fall down, remember you have a long history of getting up. Evolution might seem cold, utilitarian, or even cruel, but it's not sadistic. Disappointment is not meaningless suffering. The pain of disappointment is the attention-getting device evolution attached to a potentially life-saving message. As I said before, disappointment is a signal to adapt: *Find another way to get what you need, because whatever you're doing now isn't working.* So even while you're feeling disappointed, the need connected to your unmet expectation still waits to be satisfied. If you don't know what that need is, go back to those basic questions about your expectations: *How did I expect to feel when this expectation was met? Can I help myself feel this in other ways?* The emotion is your destination, and the expectation is the route you're going to take. Your GPS Lady is a topographical genius; she knows how to get *everywhere.*

Disappointment Helps Define Your Destination

When you've had some time to ice your bumps and bruises and you know you can be objective, revisit your disappointment and reality-test it. Reality-testing your disappointment activates and connects you to your Greatest Potential Self, because it reminds you of what you are truly seeking: a satisfied need, not a specific situation. Reality-testing your disappointment is not that different from how you reality-test your expectations. You're essentially asking yourself the same questions, only in the past tense.

Go back in your mind's eye and watch everything in slow motion. *Was I inflexible in my expectations? What was I expecting to happen? What was I expecting to feel or do? What did I expect others to feel or do? How much control, if any, did I have? What can I not do because of this outcome? What can I do only because of this outcome? Will this matter in a day? A week? A month? A year?* The answers to these questions are invaluable information, because they grant you a more lucid understanding of and perspective on your disappointment. This information allows your GPS to calibrate and adjust your unmet expectation and reorient it to satisfy your unmet need. You've figured out where *not* to go, and you're ready to try an alternate route. Punch in that new address to your inner GPS. And give yourself some credit here, because you're showing some serious guts: *You're setting new expectations while you're feeling disappointed.*

Of course, no matter how finely attuned you are to your Greatest Potential Self, or how adept you might be at communicating your expectations, people still will sometimes let you down. Like the time a pregnant client's friend promised to drive her to the hospital if she needed it. When my client went into labor and called her friend, that friend flaked because she was waiting for a mattress delivery between noon and 4:00, and it was only 3:45 (#TrueStory). That may have been the only time I've ever seen someone *murderously* disappointed. Maybe you've felt that way too. But know this: while you can't teach other people how to treat you, other people can teach you how to treat yourself (and by the way, "You Teach People How to Treat You" is also #BadAdvice). Remember: Disappointment might temporarily disconnect you from your Greatest Potential Self, but it can never push it out of reach.

Patience Is the Confidence of Knowing That What's Coming Is Better than What's Here

Healing is an automatic process, but it's never a rush job. You need time and distance to get over disappointment, and it's on you to create that psychological space for yourself. Start by cleaning house. Acknowledge and soothe your pain. Talk about it. Write about it. Reflect on it. Reality-test it. You'll gradually begin to reconnect with your Greatest Potential Self. And again, there's no rush here. You're allowed to step back, take a breath, and give yourself time to process what's going on before reaching out to talk to the person who disappointed you.

Dr. Lance Dodes is a leading figure in the treatment of addiction. He's also controversial because he questions many accepted conventions of how we treat addiction, such as making ninety twelve-step meetings in ninety days. In one interview he talked about how long it can take to break addictions. "If we could get cancer cured in eight months, we would all be happy," he says. "I don't think there's anything wrong with taking time. It always takes time." You're allowed to take time, too. Your Greatest Potential Self is worth it.

Depending on the nature of the disappointment you're dealing with, when you feel ready, you might want to talk to whoever let you down. This opens the way for empathy. And the more you make room for empathy, the less room you'll have for pain. When you don't meet your expectations of yourself and you show yourself empathy, that helps you reconnect with your Greatest Potential Self. And this can also happen when you do the same for someone else who didn't meet an expectation, leading to a wider, bird's-eye view of the situation. Maybe you miscommunicated and your expectation wasn't as clear as you thought it was. Maybe the person who let you down even has a legit reason for not meeting your expectation. And by the way, choosing a box spring delivery over a baby delivery isn't one of them.

Your Greatest Potential Self Can't Redo Yesterday, but There Are No Limits to What It Can Do with Tomorrow

As amazing as your inner GPS is, it's missing one gear: reverse. You can't undo a past disappointment, and you can't undo someone not meeting an expectation. But your Greatest Potential Self *can* decide whether you want to risk putting the same expectation on someone who didn't meet it. A sign of maturity is knowing where your expectations of certain friends have limitations. A sign of insanity is expecting the same thing from someone who has consistently failed to meet your expectation (Exhibit A: the irresponsible fuckup who ate the Talenti ice cream).

Whether or not you talk to the person who disappointed you, and whether or not you change your expectations of them, *you must forgive them*. Even if the other person fucked up so bad that you never want to see them again, you can still forgive them. They don't have to know. Forgiving someone doesn't mean you excuse or justify whatever they did or didn't do. You can absolutely forgive someone for wrecking your car without ever handing them your keys again. This said, you don't suddenly have amnesia regarding the accident. You proceed with knowledge. NOT caution, NOT forgetfulness, NOT denial. Forgiveness is self-empowerment; *it empowers you to move into the future, not to undo the past*.

I have a black belt in forgiveness: My assistant crashed my car, and I forgave her AND gave her the keys again. So I'm either a Jesus-Level Forgiver . . . or I'm stupid. (You don't have to choose right now.) By forgiving someone, you make a conscious choice to direct your energy toward recovering from disappointment instead of reminding yourself of who caused it. Forgiveness is a process. It doesn't always happen all at once, and you don't need to rush it. Have faith in your ability to forgive, even if you can't do it right away.

Being open to forgiveness also reconnects you to your GPS, because your Greatest Potential Self is just that, your *Potential* self. It's the best possible version of you, the version of you in the future who's already forgiven the person who let you down. Like the future version of my formerly pregnant client who already forgave her friend for flaking on her promise.

The Expectations of Your Greatest Potential Self Lead to Your Greatest Present Self

The #BadAdvice of *Expectations Lead to Disappointment* is a lie of omission. Yes, expectations lead to disappointment, but they lead to so much more as well. Your expectations help you to satisfy your needs and find meaning, connection, fulfillment, and infinitely more in life. This happens because your expectations connect you with the guidance offered by your Greatest Potential Self, and that connection is made through your emotions. Denying disappointment, or any emotion, breaks that connection. Being tuned in to your inner GPS means you're able to recognize disappointment as part of your navigational system. You accept the potential for pain, because you know that pain carries a benefit with it. That benefit is a clearer understanding of yourself, your needs, and how you can meet those needs. Recognizing this truth frees you from fearing disappointment and helps you find the courage to embrace your expectations. Expectations lead beyond disappointment. They lead you to your Greatest Potential Self.

EXPECTATIONS LEAD TO YOUR GPS:
GREATEST POTENTIAL SELF
#GOODADVICE

4

YOU GET WHAT YOU GET
AND YOU DON'T GET UPSET

Telling someone *You Get What You Get and You Don't Get Upset* is such a barefaced and demeaning message of disempowerment that it would seem ridiculous used between adults. That's why we save it for kids. This little gem is straight off the #BadAdvice Kids' Menu, usually heard in elementary schools and playgrounds across America.

I realize that overworked, underpaid teachers aren't intentionally dispensing it, but this #BadAdvice is the language of oppression set to a Mother Goose rhyme scheme. The people who pass on this advice probably heard or saw it in another classroom and thought, "Aww, what a cute way to tell a kid to shut the fuck up."

When I was researching this chapter, I found articles and parenting blogs that extolled the "wisdom" of this #BadAdvice. They claimed that teaching kids to get what they get and not get upset somehow instilled a sense of gratitude. But this #BadAdvice doesn't teach gratitude. For one thing, research shows that the brain's ability to experience gratitude develops between the ages of seven and ten, long after preschool. So it isn't about instilling gratitude. It's about enforcing submission to the status quo. *You Get What You Get and You Don't Get Upset* warns you that how you feel and what you need do not matter when they're an inconvenience to Authority.

Even if you've never been told *You Get What You Get and You Don't Upset*, you've heard some version of it. *Don't be a crybaby. Keep crying and I'll give you something to cry about. You're too sensitive.* Or the brutally simple, *Stop crying.* Crying is no different from laughing—an immediate and involuntary emotional release. What you are really being told is *Your suffering is an inconvenience.*

When you hear this message over and over, you begin to believe that what you need and what you want don't matter. So you shut up and accept whatever's given to you. It's like being told, "I'm going to smack you; don't you dare say ouch." This #BadAdvice originates from a place of inequality, and the unequal power distribution between adults and children is why we get away with telling this shit to kids. If you went around telling other adults to get what they get and not get upset, you'd get smacked with a bag of nickels.

"This isn't what I ordered."

"YOU GET WHAT YOU GET AND YOU DON'T
GET UPSET."

"That's not my prescription."

"YOU GET WHAT YOU GET AND YOU DON'T
GET UPSET."

"You don't go down on me anymore."

"YOU GET WHAT YOU GET AND YOU DON'T
GET UPSET."

Right? It sounds ridiculous in an adult context. But *You Get What You Get and You Don't Get Upset* is a slogan of toxic authority that still plays out in the adult world. Kids may hear it the most, but the same #BadAdvice that denies needs and feelings in the classroom or the playground denies rights and freedoms in the world. It's #OppressiveAdvice, on a global scale. *You Get What You Get and You Don't Get Upset* is how Old Power responds to the force of New Change. If you're a woman, don't expect equal pay for equal work: *You Get What You Get and You Don't Get Upset*. Don't expect acceptance for your sinful LGBTQIA lifestyle: *You Get What You Get and You Don't Get Upset*. Black Lives Don't Matter, because *You Get What You Get and You Don't Get Upset* . . . and so on.

I'm not the only one who sees this connection. After the Women's March in January 2017, Dina Leygerman, a writer for the parenting website Romper, wrote a response to those who denied that sexism still exists in America: "You believe feminists are emotional, irrational, unreasonable. Why aren't women just satisfied with their lives, right? You get what you get and you don't get upset, right?" But, hey, I get it. Familiarity makes even the most toxic dysfunction feel normal, even comfortable. The voice of authority makes that dysfunction *unquestionable*. Especially when it comes from the Highest Authority.

All This Religion Is Giving God a Bad Name

One of the earliest versions of *You Get What You Get and You Don't Get Upset* is in the New Testament, in the book of Matthew: *Blessed are the meek, for they shall inherit the earth*. But it's not the #ChristAdvice that's #BadAdvice. In the Bible, the word "meek" is the common translation for the Greek word *praus*. But *praus* does *not* mean meek; according to one concordance, it means "exercising strength under God's control, i.e., demonstrating power without undue harshness." Translating *praus* as merely "meek" transforms a message of gentle power into one of submissiveness.

This may not have been entirely coincidental. American theologian Mark Y. A. Davies pointed out that "once the [Roman] Empire co-opted the Christian movement, it focused on the otherworldly aspects of Christianity in order to keep power and control over people in this world." In other words, "Accept your shitty life, because after you die everything will be awesome forever, we promise." *You Get What You Get and You Don't Get Upset* is a newer version of some very old machinery of oppression. The ancient Romans are long gone, but they left that machinery running on their way out. Fast forward a few thousand years. Here you are, living in a society that conditions you to deny your own needs, the needs of other people, and the pain of those needs going unmet. But for as tough and long-lasting as this #BadAdvice has been, *you* have access to something greater, and it's already within you.

Instincts: The Built-In Security System Too Many of Us Choose to Ignore

In every one of your cells, you carry an intuitive wisdom stretching back to prehistory, a survival guide hardwired into you at birth. Science calls this wisdom *instinct*. One medium through which your instincts communicate with you is your emotions. Emotions evolved as part of your biological survival gear. When you experience an emotion, your brain's limbic system sends chemical messages to the rest of your body, creating the physical experience of that emotion. The limbic system is a primitive part of your brain. Its job is to handle primal urges, like eating, fucking, and not becoming lunch for a cave bear. So while you can exercise *some* control over your emotions, there is no master control switch. Which means the #BadAdvice of *You Get What You Get and You Don't Get Upset* is also #ImpossibleAdvice, because this #BadAdvice *rejects science*. It's climate change denial on the personal level. Ignore your emotions, and you ignore your biology. That's a very dangerous thing.

What do your emotions have to do with your survival? According to studies led by Dr. Rachael E. Jack at the University of Glasgow, it's all over your face. Your eyes going wide in fear is a biological adaptation to try to get more visual information about a frightening situation so you can more effectively deal with it. Scrunching up your face in disgust is designed to shield your nose from breathing in anything harmful coming off whatever's grossing you out. And your prehistoric ancestors' facial expressions in moments like these would have alerted others to the danger.

Your emotions are as much a part of your biology as your psychology. They are an enduring survival adaptation of our evolution, and evolution doesn't commit to mistakes (although given human history, we might second-guess its success). Emotions are a lot like your physical senses: They translate your experiences into messages for your brain to process and act on. You can't decide not to feel something any more than you can decide not to smell something, as appealing as either of those impossible options may be. And by the way, *your emotions are not the same thing as your feelings*.

Think about how you can physically *feel* your face flush when something embarrassing happens; or the lead-heavy, tangible weight you feel in your chest when someone breaks your heart; or the adrenaline rush of fear. Those are all the physical *feelings* of embarrassment, heartbreak, and fear. You experience their corresponding emotions once your brain processes the physiological sensation. The #BadAdvice of *You Get What You Get and You Don't Get Upset* puts a lock on that process. You can't figure out how you feel or what to do about it *if you deny how you feel.* Your emotions are messengers carrying potential life-saving information about yourself and your surroundings. Ignoring them is like ignoring the fire alarm in a burning building.

Too Many of Us Choose Fear Over Being Free

Disappointment, anger, frustration, sadness, fear, and any other version of "getting upset" are emotional experiences of unmet needs. *You Get What You Get and You Don't Get Upset* does nothing to help you when your needs go unmet. When your paycheck is smaller because of your gender, when you're confronted with hate speech, when anyone dismisses your worth and fulfillment as a human being—all this #BadAdvice has to add is, *Yeah, take that. You Get What You Get and You Don't Get Upset, Bitch.*

This same dynamic plays out on the macro scale. All too often, *You Get What You Get and You Don't Get Upset* is society's answer to the collective pain of people's unmet needs for freedom, dignity, and respect. And it's those times when people like Emma González and Martin Luther King Jr. step forward to show people just how much power there is in *getting upset*. But you can't tap into the power of being upset if you deny the feeling to begin with. And if you deny your feelings, you can't satisfy the need (or needs) behind those feelings. So are you really going to surrender your right to satisfy your needs and obey the idiot law of this #BadAdvice? *Fuck no.* You're going to follow this chapter's #GoodAdvice.

If What You Need's Not What You Get, You Better Fucking Get Upset #GOODADVICE

Another reason this #BadAdvice makes my head explode is rooted in my hometown. Upper Darby, Pennsylvania, is a blue-collar suburb of Philadelphia. It's where my parents raised my three sisters, my brother, and myself in a house that barely had room for the seven of us, and *no* room for bullshit like *You Get What You Get and You Don't Get Upset*. In fact, the received wisdom in Upper Darby was that if you weren't getting what you needed, *then you got off your ass and fought for it.* (Then again, I'm white. Not everyone gets cut the same break as me when they defy authority.) We weren't taught to deny what we felt. We learned to express it in some fucked-up, destructive ways, but we didn't deny it. *You Get What You Get, Then You Torch That Asshole's Fucking Car.*

Part of what makes this #BadAdvice such a mindfuck is that while it denies what you feel, it cultivates *other* emotions within you. It helps you feel unworthy and afraid. Denying your emotions reinforces the idea that you are unworthy of satisfying your needs. Fear comes with this #BadAdvice because like all toxic authoritative messages, it carries an implied threat of *"or else!"* They are statements of intimidation. *Fuck them.* You can't choose whether or not you get upset about something, but you don't have to be afraid. You don't. You also don't have to fear the power already within you— the power to move past fear and change your corner of the world.

It Doesn't Matter If You're Afraid; What Matters Is What Your Fear Drives You to Do

Nearly any fear can feel as terrifying as death itself because, well, according to the ancient part of your brain, *it is*. Part of the limbic system is the amygdala. Among other things, the amygdala manages fear. But surrounding your primitive brain is your neocortex, which is where you'll find most of the awesome software upgrades made by evolution like language, emotional processing, and being able to persuade the doctor you have a legitimate need for a weed prescription.

The thing is, your brain's function is the result of these and other neural systems all working together simultaneously. Your neocortex's risk assessment of a situation might be, *He's gonna be pissed when I ask for the Nespresso machine he stole from me when he moved out.* But your limbic system's read on what's going on is *HOLY SHIT WE'RE GONNA DIE GET US THE FUCK OUTTA HERE!* Your amygdala sends out the Fight, Flight, or Freeze signal. The mind and body immediately release chemicals and hormones preparing you to either *fight* off the threat, take *flight* to escape, or *freeze* and try to hide. When your sophisticated neocortex receives that message in a scary, but not deadly, situation, it translates *Fight, Flight, or Freeze* to the less-urgent *Fuck It* response. Your misperceived fear becomes a misguided survival impulse, and you actively avoid those things you should be seeking: *You deliberately block yourself from meeting your needs.* If you've ever seen someone self-sabotage, procrastinate, or suggest "Maybe we should give him a chance" after the 2016 election, you've seen the freeze response to fear. Even so, fear is not your enemy. It's an emotion that evolved to help keep you alive, not to keep you from living.

The #BadAdvice of *You Get What You Get and You Don't Get Upset* hides the truth of how you feel and what you need behind an illusion of fear. You may need some courage to remind yourself that fear is an obstacle, not an authority. Which is okay, because you are capable of courage. Unlike this #BadAdvice, finding courage doesn't start with denying what you feel. Courage begins when you admit you're afraid.

Decide You're More Courageous Than Afraid

"Courage" is a loaded word. It's one of those words like "honor," "loyalty," or "Gucci" that sounds like it should be chiseled into marble somewhere. We usually use the word "courage" in the context of mind-blowing heroism. But courage isn't just the stuff of stories and history books, and it's not as rare as you may think. Being courageous doesn't mean being unafraid. Any idiot can take a risk without thinking about it: The continued existence of Las Vegas depends on it. *Real* courage is understanding that no matter how scary a risk might seem, *not taking the risk is scarier.*

You already know this: Every cruel bastard you've ever stood up to, every intimidating job interview you showed up for, every nervous first date you went on, and anything else you faced down with a pounding heart and sweaty palms are proof of your courage. The word "courage" comes from *cor*, the Latin word for "heart." *That* is where your courage, and all courage, comes from. When you decide that love is stronger than fear, it is. Which means when you decide that *you* are stronger than fear, you are. So how do you do this? Give yourself permission to be afraid. Because when you give yourself permission to be afraid, *you also give yourself permission to be courageous.*

Your primal fear response comes with a manual override switch: *you.* In a scientific experiment, volunteers with a fear of snakes were placed next to a conveyor belt with a snake on it and told to hit a button that would move the snake closer to them. When participants decided to move the snake closer, brain scans revealed that another part of their limbic system, the subgenual anterior cingulate cortex, *overrode the fear signal coming from the amygdala*. But this reaction only happened *after* a person hit the button to bring the snake closer. It was courage that triggered the fear-overriding response, not the other way around. The switch won't flip if you're following this #BadAdvice and pretending not to be upset. Get upset, feel afraid, then choose to be courageous. Courage is the feeling of being effectively afraid. This is something you can practice.

You can start by doing one thing each day that scares you. (But be safe, not stupid.) Ask for a raise. Stop settling for boring sex. Call your member of Congress and tell him or her what to do. Tell someone you love them. Call bullshit on sexism and racism when you see it. Be the person who steps in and helps when everyone else is just standing by. Tell your mom you're staying at a hotel this Christmas. Facing and experiencing fear creates indisputable proof that it won't destroy you, and more important, it proves your potential for courage. The decision to be courageous is instantly transformative and undeniably real. What was once the source of your fear becomes a source of new information and understanding. When you give the #BadAdvice of *You Get What You Get and You Don't Get Upset* the boot and have the courage to *Get Upset*, you empower yourself to be *effectively afraid*. Instead of freezing in fear, *you take action in spite of it*.

Sometimes Getting What You Need Is Scary: It Can Remind You of Every Time You Didn't

Before you face your fear, you need to be sure you can recognize it. When unfaced fear is your constant companion, it often camouflages itself as another emotion. Anger, pessimism, cynicism, even boredom are all potential masks of fear. Do you consistently associate these kinds of feelings with certain people or situations?

Your fear could also be working undercover. The #BadAdvice of *You Get What You Get and You Don't Get Upset* keeps fear hidden, because it keeps you in denial of it. Your courage changes that. Instead of hiding from your fear, *you fucking challenge it until it backs down*. Once you've faced your fear, you can get curious about the unmet needs behind it. You can finally ask yourself, *What do I need?*

So? What *do* you need? Can you even answer that question? Do you have a need for stability? Do you need excitement? Intimacy? Acceptance? Connection? Do you need to express yourself? To be recognized? *What do I need?* As your needs reveal themselves to you, follow up by asking, *Am I meeting this need? If so, do I meet it in a way that's positive or negative? What does it create in my life? How does it affect other people?* How do you even know when you're meeting a need? You'll know because *you'll feel fucking great*.

Studies show that each one of your individual needs creates a unique sensation of well-being when it's satisfied. Think back to the last time you felt *really* good—so good that you could describe it as a feeling of *intense well-being*. Whatever you did to arrive at that feeling of intense well-being is a way you met your needs. Maybe you have a memory of feeling spectacular in a moment of achievement. That feeling was an experience of satisfying your need for accomplishment. I can guarantee that in that moment, you were not following this chapter's #BadAdvice. *You Get What You Get and You Don't Get Upset* will never help you feel anything positive, because it will never help you meet a single need.

On top of that, *You Get What You Get and You Don't Get Upset* is #BadAdvice with a #DoubleEdge, because your needs don't stop with you. New research shows that people tend to be happier when the needs of others in their society are also fulfilled. So another one of your needs is helping others get what they need. It's not just the person hearing this #BadAdvice who's cut off from how they feel and what they need: *Dispensing this bullshit disrupts your own need to help others.* Finding fulfillment and meeting your needs is not a solo gig, so don't be afraid to open doors for others (both the figurative and literal kind). You can open a door for someone else and still walk through it after them.

Ignoring Pain Is Like Ignoring a Fire Alarm

As a culture, we try to prepare for all kinds of emergencies, except the emotional ones. This blows my mind, given our

obsession with emergencies: Fire alarms. Emergency exits.
Fire escape routes posted on hotel room doors. Adults being
instructed on the complex mechanics of an airline seatbelt.
When shit's on fire, you're handed a fire extinguisher. But
when *you're* on fire with the pain of an unmet need, you're
handed #BadAdvice: *You Get What You Get and You Don't Get
Upset.* Not anymore. It's time to do for yourself what no one
else can: *Arm yourself with the know-how of how to Get Upset.*

Feelings Come and Go, but the People You're Connected to Remain

Who are the people you call when you get upset? During an
Emotional 9–1–1, who can you depend on to remind you of
everything you are outside of the moment you're in? Who can
best help you see yourself as a whole? Don't hesitate to lean on
those you're closest to when you need them. The #BadAdvice
of *You Get What You Get and You Don't Get Upset* makes it
seem like your needs, your emotions, and by extension *you*
aren't important enough to bother anyone with.

Bullshit. You're allowed to be your own strongest advo-
cate. Ask for help, and help will come. How can I be so sure?
The people who care about you, wait for it . . . *care about you.*
You are important to them. *Ask for help when you need it.*

Real Life: Available Everywhere in HD with Surround Sound

Alright, all this stuff about needs and emotions is great, but
what about some *immediate pain relief?* How can you calm

your emotional ocean after you recognize that you're upset? You probably don't need me to tell you that changing your environment, getting outside, and just moving can help you feel better in the moment. And if you're hurting right now, I'm sure "Take a walk!" sounds like #DumbAssAdvice. But the specifics of what you do to relieve your pain in the moment matter less than your awareness of *why* you're doing it. You can give your actions a deeper meaning, and that deeper meaning has a deeper effect.

A good friend of mine takes a specific bike route when she needs relief, and she almost always feels better at the end of her ride. The familiarity of the scenery, the physicality of riding the bike, and the sensation of moving all help break the circuit and redirect her energy. A stress-reducing practice developed in Japan known as *shinrin-yoku* (forest bathing) involves nothing more than finding a nice quiet spot in the woods or somewhere similar and . . . doing nothing and relaxing. But doing nothing *on purpose* can actually do a lot: Studies show that *shinrin-yoku* can lower blood pressure and levels of the stress hormone, cortisol. So forget that #BadAdvice that tells you *Don't Get Upset. Get Upset!* And after you get upset . . . *go outside.*

A Great Song Is a Wake-up Call for Your Soul

You can find good medicine in music. I'm serious about this, and so is the science. Multiple studies link listening to mellow music with mellow emotions. Listening to slower-tempo music can also reduce the level of cortisol in your system. Surgery patients even reported a decrease in *physical* pain after listening to music.

But let's be clear, it takes more than a brisk walk and slow jamz on your earbuds to help you feel better. Easing pain doesn't mean eliminating it. And that's a good thing. For as much as emotional pain sucks, it almost always brings you a message you need to hear: *You're not getting what you need.* That's a message you can't receive when the #BadAdvice of *You Get What You Get and You Don't Get Upset* is screening your calls.

No Matter How Lonely You Feel, You Are Never Alone

"Getting upset" is not a permanent condition, and neither are any of your emotions. What and how you feel is always shifting and changing. But what if that doesn't feel true for you? What if instead of moving on its natural currents and tides, your emotional ocean is flat, cold, and still? That's how I describe depression: It's a pause in someone's emotional pulse.

Medical science, and people in general, don't understand a lot about depression yet. The pain of clinical depression can be agonizing, and it can be beyond explanation for those who've never known it firsthand. But the mental health community (industry) has so overpathologized normal human emotions that the average person has a hard time distinguishing between being legitimately upset and being clinically depressed. What we do know for sure is that clinical depression is not a character defect or a sign of weakness. And it is nothing anyone should be expected to handle alone.

If any of this hits home with you, put this book down now and call someone. Talk to that person. Without knowing a thing about you, I can promise you this: *You are needed and loved.* If the pain is unbearable, you can talk to someone 24–7 at the National Suicide Prevention Lifeline at 1–800–273–TALK (8255). And I totally get it if the idea of talking to someone feels too overwhelming. You can still find support through the Crisis Text Line. Text HOME to 741741 in the US, or to 686868 in Canada. Someone who cares and is ready to help you will respond.

There Is No Better Story than One You Don't Know the End Of

You are in a constant state of change and motion. Cells divide, hair and fingernails lengthen imperceptibly, the electric impulses of your thoughts rocket around your brain at warp speed. For as real and verifiable as all of that is, it probably doesn't figure in to how you see yourself, because cells, hair, fingernails, and thoughts go about their business silent and unseen. What *does* immediately inform your sense of self are those things you *are* aware of, especially your emotions. *You Get What You Get and You Don't Get Upset* distorts your sense of self: Denying what you feel stops you from seeing your whole, true self. Which means that the ongoing, told-in-real-time story you tell yourself about you, something psychologists call your *personal narrative*, isn't true to who you really are.

Everyone has both positive and negative self-narratives, and these narratives run in our heads all day, every day. You might have a negative personal narrative about your job, a positive personal narrative about being single, a negative personal narrative around the ever-present nagging feeling that you could be getting more from life, and narratives everywhere in between about all the other shit you have going on. Your emotions and your needs inform these narratives. Which is why denying how you feel or what you need blinds you to the truth of who you really are. Getting upset when you don't get what you need helps keep that truth in focus. Sooooooo . . . *Get Upset!*

Get Upset. Your emotions are powerful catalysts for change in your life. *Get Upset.* What matters most about your personal narratives is that you realize they, like you, are always changing. You are never fixed in your existence. You may not always know in every moment how, why, and what you feel or need. But you never need to fear any of it. For as much as it changes, your narrative endures as something that is exclusively *yours*. *Get Upset.* When you submit to the #BadAdvice of *You Get What You Get and You Don't Get Upset*, you surrender your authority over your personal narrative. And that is like trading a palace for a prison cell.

On the Other Side of Every Struggle
Waits a Greater Version of Who You Are Now

Per aspera ad astra—Latin for "through adversity to the stars"—is the motto of many police departments, cities, fire departments, and universities the world over. One of the reasons it's so popular with groups like these is that *it's a reminder of the human potential for courage.* Since you're a human, this includes you.

A lot of self-help writers and thinkers seem to assume that everyone in their audience already exists in a Fully Realized Superhuman state. *You're already fearless and powerful; you just forgot. Good thing I reminded you (you're welcome).* This drives me batshit insane. Even Fully Realized Superhumans don't feel great all the time. Not only are you allowed to feel bad, but sometimes you *need* to feel bad before you can get what you need. It's why the potential for courage is hard-wired into you—*because you need it.*

Sometimes you won't get what you want. Or sometimes you'll get what you want, only to discover it doesn't satisfy you the way you thought it would. Sometimes, even when you understand your feelings and know what you need, satisfying your needs will be difficult, scary, painful, and who knows what else. But you won't remain afraid. Instead of trying to deny or escape your unmet needs and the fear and pain surrounding them, you'll acknowledge and engage with all of it. You'll decide to be more courageous than afraid. You'll transcend fear and reveal your feelings, along with the needs connected to them. You'll recognize how those emotions and needs connect you with others. You'll remember your undeniable worth, because you *are* worthy. You are worthy of all you feel, and every one of your needs is worthy of satisfaction. Once you know this, you become a champion of your own truth. The truth of what you feel. The truth of what you need. The truth of who you are. And of course, the truth of this #GoodAdvice:

IF WHAT YOU NEED IS NOT WHAT YOU GET,
YOU BETTER FUCKING GET UPSET
#GOODADVICE

5

NOBODY CAN MAKE YOU FEEL BAD WITHOUT YOUR PERMISSION

Nobody Can Make You Feel Bad Without Your Permission means, in other words, *If you're hurting, you fucked up.* That's more than #BadAdvice. It's a #BigLie.

This message ranks with some of the biggest lies you've been told, like *You Will Use Algebra as an Adult, You Might Feel Some Slight Discomfort,* and *They're All the Same Size When Erect. Nobody Can Make You Feel Bad Without Your Permission* is the #BadAdvice you hear when other people hurt you. You can't pick and choose which emotions you want to feel, because emotions never ask permission. But this #BadAdvice expects you to believe that insults, hate speech, and emotional abuse hurt only if you decide to "opt in." In other words, *If you're hurting, you fucked up. Nobody*

Can Make You Feel Bad Without Your Permission is *Sticks and Stones May Break My Bones but Names Will Never Hurt Me* in grown-up clothing.

But no matter what this #BadAdvice is wearing when you hear it, it disintegrates the second it's reality tested. Would you say this shit to a woman who's slut-shamed on the internet? Or a gay kid who found "FAGGOT" written on his locker? Or a black person who was just called the N-word? And if words have no power to harm, why did I feel the need to write "the N-word" just now, instead of *that* word? Because the idea that what other people say and do has no power to affect how you feel is bullshit.

"Nobody Can Make You Feel Bad Without Your Permission" Was Probably Said by Someone Who Was Never Abused and Is a Load of Shit

Nobody Can Make You Feel Bad Without Your Permission is a form of psychological abuse known as *gaslighting*. Gaslighting happens at both the cultural and interpersonal levels. It can be as complex and far reaching as a propaganda campaign, or as brutally simple as an abuser's rejection of facts: *I never hit you. I never said that. It's all in your head. It's Fake News!* Gaslighting is a deliberate, ongoing process of denial, deceit, and deception. The term comes from a 1938 British play called *Gas Light* (and two movies made in the 1940s), in which a woman is subjected to this kind of abuse. Gaslighting is crazy-making behavior at its darkest because it makes you doubt your own memory, reality, and sanity.

So along with being #BadAdvice and a #BigLie, telling people *Nobody Can Make You Feel Bad Without Your Permission* is abusive. It says that the hurt you feel is your responsibility, not that of the person who has hurt you. Your pain isn't real, because it doesn't exist outside you. You chose it; it's all in your head.

Sticks and Stones May Break Bones, but Words Can Do Some Serious Fucking Damage

Who gives a shit about sticks, stones, and breaking bones? Broken bones heal. But the same can't be said for brain damage. I'm dead fuck'n serious: *Verbal and emotional abuse can cause actual brain damage.* The corpus callosum is a dense collection of nerve fibers linking the right and left sides of your brain. Brain scans of adults who were bullied in middle school revealed an underdeveloped corpus callosum: Their brains were underconnected. The same group of people struggled with anxiety, depression, anger, hostility, dissociation, and drug abuse. And by the way, *none of these people came from abusive homes.* The cruelty of a few asshole kids in middle school was potent enough to cause brain damage. I can promise you that not one of the people in this study gave anyone permission to fuck up their brains. *Nobody Can Make You Feel Bad Without Your Permission?* Fuck right off with that.

You're Not Responsible for How Other People Help You Feel, but You Can Choose What You Want Help Feeling

Nobody Can Make You Feel Bad Without Your Permission finds fault in the very stuff that makes you human. Because while it's true that nobody can literally *make* you feel a certain way, people can definitely *influence* and *inspire* the emotions you experience. That's a good thing. Our ability to inspire emotions in each other is a built-in guarantee that the human species keeps improving. It's often the mechanism that drives yet another evolutionary survival adaptation: cooperation. As a species, we are both socially emotional and emotionally social. It's what made us the evolutionary success story we are (okay, a *qualified* success: We lose points for inventing war, pollution, and toddler beauty pageants). Emotions exist for a reason: Evolution doesn't commit to mistakes. The emotions we inspire in each other are not symptoms of weakness or personal failings. We are chemically designed to connect with each other.

One of those chemical connections happens through the hormone and neurotransmitter oxytocin. Oxytocin can nurture feelings of generosity, trust, and connection. It can even facilitate physical healing. A primary release trigger for oxytocin *is the way another person helps you feel*. Your brain releases oxytocin whenever you hug someone, experience an affectionate touch, have sex, or even just share a laugh with another person. Because of these positive social triggers, oxytocin is often called "the love hormone." But that's not accurate, *because love isn't the only emotion that triggers oxytocin's release.*

Researchers have found that negative emotions like sadness and hate can also elicit a release of oxytocin in your brain. There's also anecdotal evidence suggesting that interacting with people on social media is yet another stimulus for an oxytocin hit. So the same powerful chemical that bonds friends and lovers also bonds the Klansmen at a crossburning or an online mob of cyberbullies. I'll assume you're not a member of the Klan or a cyberbully (if you are, your problems exceed the scope of this book), but you still need to be conscious of not only who you're connecting with, but how you feel in that connection.

You won't access that awareness trying to follow the #BadAdvice of *Nobody Can Make You Feel Bad Without Your Permission,* because it denies that anyone can help anyone else feel anything. Worse than just #BadAdvice and a #BigLie, it's #DangerousAdvice. But if this #BadAdvice is so crazy-making, dangerous, and clearly untrue, why do we keep repeating it? Because *Nobody Can Make You Feel Bad Without Your Permission* tempts you with an impossible-to-deliver-on promise. It tries to sell you on the idea that someone can hurt you only if you agree to it. It denies more than emotional and psychological truth; *it denies biological truth.* You, like every other person in the world, are emotionally, psychologically, and biochemically connected with the people around you. And sometimes those people will help you feel bad, because just like your emotions, *conflict in life is inevitable*. So this #BadAdvice promises you more than a place to hide from your emotional pain; *it dupes you into thinking you can escape conflict*.

Cardboard Conflict vs. Concrete Conflict

We live in an age of Conflict Culture. From reality TV to national politics, "winning," "losing," and choosing a "side" matter more than ideas, or even reality. Arguing with strangers online is the video game we can all agree on. All of this bullshit combines to create the ultimate product of Conflict Culture, something I call *Cardboard Conflict*. Just like cardboard, Cardboard Conflict is cheap and easy to shape into whatever we want, and we recycle the shit out of it. It's not even always bad. People have always lapped up conflict as entertainment. (Shit, I wouldn't be on TV without it!) A story with no conflict would be pretty fucking boring. Nobody watches the Super Bowl to see the two teams share the ball and play nice. But what you don't find in Cardboard Conflict is any kind of guide to resolving the real, *concrete conflicts* you face in life.

It's hard not to get stuck in a headspace of perpetual and aggressive disagreement when you're buried alive in the bullshit messages of Conflict Culture. You might learn how to ape the motions of outrage, but you'll have no clue how to move past the fight or get closer in your personal relationships.

When you don't know how to resolve the concrete conflicts in your own life, you hide from them. But the feelings the conflicts stirred up are still there. So you try to find another way to purge those feelings, a behavior psychology calls *sublimation*. Maybe you get angry or go into denial. Or maybe you try to lose yourself in some Cardboard Conflict. If this is something you do, it's nothing to be embarrassed about. You can't expect yourself to resolve conflict if the only guide you have for it is the #BadAdvice that *Nobody Can Make You Feel Bad Without Your Permission*.

The word "conflict" comes with a bad rep and heavy baggage. It's used to describe anything from a personal disagreement to a full-blown fucking war. But whether it's a conflict between wild animals, a couple sitting on the opposite ends of my couch during a session, or two countries arguing over the size and power of their nuclear buttons, the core dynamic of a conflict is always the same: A conflict is the result of unmet needs. Like when too many animals show up at the same watering hole: Somebody's going home thirsty. North Korea's need to be respected as a world power conflicts with everyone else's need not to be blown the fuck up. My editor's need for the final draft of this chapter conflicted with my need to binge-watch *Game of Thrones*.

You can see from these examples why we usually associate the idea of conflict with anger, frustration, and aggression— you know, the way you felt last month, last week, or maybe yesterday. *The way you feel when somebody makes you feel bad without your permission*. You didn't give them permission, and you sure as shit don't need anyone's permission to do something about it. It's on you to put things in motion, resolve your conflict, and help yourself feel better. No one else can do it. *You* have the final call over what you think, what you say, how you act and how you respond to everyone and everything. Which brings me to my #GoodAdvice.

You Were Born a Boss #GOODADVICE

I mean it. *You were born a boss.* You're not the boss of everything all the time, but you are *always* the Boss of You. Being the Boss of You is your lifetime gig. There will never be anyone on this planet more qualified for this job than you. All the components and processes of your heart, mind, and body form an organization that has a single purpose: *to create and sustain your existence and the existence of others.* Your emotions, your thoughts, your needs—they all ultimately serve *you.* You. Are. The. Boss. You're the Boss and *that's your fucking job.*

And since you're the Boss, you can't hide in your office when a conflict jams up your life's assembly line. You can't ignore it and hope it will go away. You can't wait for someone else to fix it, because you're the one who needs to do the fixing. The Boss knows that *Nobody Can Make You Feel Bad Without Your Permission* is bullshit, because *a conflict never asks permission.* And the Boss never asks permission to find resolution.

Bosses Don't Avoid Conflict;
They See It as Opportunity

As the Boss, you know your business better than anyone else. So when someone helps you feel bad, you know it's a sign that you're in conflict with that person, not that you fucked up. And when you know that behind every conflict is a collision of unmet needs, you know what to do next: Check in with your needs and emotions. You're the Boss, so ask for a status report. *How do I feel right now? Who or what helped me feel this way? Why do I feel unsatisfied? What can I do to change this? What do I need?* Conflict is upsetting for anyone, but there's also an emotion only Bosses like you can find in it: *motivation.* A Boss knows that avoiding conflict means avoiding opportunity, because every conflict offers opportunity. More than just being *able* to face and resolve conflict, you're *motivated* to do it.

So now, envision yourself: There you are, the Boss of You, Inc., sitting in your badass office in your ergonomic desk chair. You sip your organic fair trade chai latte from your BEST FUCKING BOSS EVER mug. Then a text comes in on your Boss Phone: *Someone just helped you feel like shit. What're you gonna do about it, Boss?* In real life, that text takes the form of emotional distress, aka "Feeling Bad." So resolving a conflict begins with giving yourself some emotional relief. *Nobody Can Make You Feel Bad Without Your Permission* is useless here, because nobody needs your permission to help you feel anything. Lucky for you, *you don't need permission to Take a Beat.*

When You Don't Like How You're Feeling, Take a Beat to Reconsider What You're Doing

Wisdom has a habit of arriving with unexpected messengers. The best advice I've ever received came from my heroin-addicted sister and best friend. Think of her as the Oracle at Delphi dispensing wisdom after inhaling white oleander fumes. (Note: I dispense this advice to you without the help of heroin or fumes, white oleander or otherwise.)

When I was in my late teens and twenties, I was passionate and explosive about the world. But under that fire and rebellion was a deep sense of powerlessness. I felt controlled by other people and my emotions. When someone helped me feel bad, I didn't know what to do. *I felt powerless because I couldn't resolve conflict.* To try to take back my power in a conflict, I'd say or do something extreme, drastic, stupid, or all three without thinking it through. Then shit would blow up in my face and I'd feel powerless again. So I'd act without thinking, shit would blow up in my face, rinse and repeat. I remember seething about something, ready to pull the pin on another grenade and throw it, when my younger sister said to me: "When people talk to you, you feel like you have to answer them right away; but you can take as long as you want to reply. Your life-time belongs to you."

My sister told me then what I'm telling you now: *You're a Boss, so You Answer on Your Own Time.* When you're not sure of anything, when you don't know what to do, when you're too upset to process what's happening around you, don't take any #BadAdvice on "feeling bad." Take a Beat, instead.

Taking a Beat starts with *self-soothing:* Talk yourself off the fucking ledge. Give yourself the relief you need. You need time and distance to recover and adjust your perspective. Give that to yourself and *step back from the conflict*. Notice I said "step back," not "run away." You're not avoiding the conflict; you're giving yourself whatever space you need. Stepping back isn't running away.

So when your finger is hovering over the "Send" button that will drop the Nuclear Bomb of Fury on that asshole who pissed you off . . . Take a Beat. Slow your roll. Give it twenty-four hours and see whether you still want to send it (and if you do, give it *another* twenty-four hours). Don't confuse this with "ghosting" someone or using passive-aggressive silence. You're the Boss; you have more class than that. Telling someone "Hey I need to take a break from this and give myself time and distance to gain a greater perspective—hold please" is proactive. You're allowed to Take a Beat and step back because you're the Boss. And the Boss doesn't just know when to step back: The Boss knows when to step back in.

Avoiding the Existing Conflict Only Creates More Conflict

It can feel counterintuitive to step back in because we want to avoid pain and discomfort, which could be why a lot of people's knee-jerk response is to avoid conflict. But the Boss knows that avoiding conflict creates more conflict. So when you feel cooled off, step back in to the conflict.

Stepping back in begins with a conversation. Let the other person know you want to cooperate and find a resolution. It's so easy during a conflict to undercommunicate about the issue, because both parties are looking to avoid discomfort and pain. Everyone's scared. Except the Boss. The Boss isn't scared of conflict. The Boss sees this kind of conversation for what it really is: *an excavation*. Even though your first impulse might be to undercommunicate, the only way out of this is to overcommunicate. *You have to keep digging.* Somewhere buried under your conflict is the resolution. It's not always easy. It won't always feel good. Sometimes it will outright suck. But I know you can handle it. *You're the Boss.* Keep the conversation going, and you'll reveal the resolution. You don't need anyone's permission to clock out or clock back in. Even if you have to keep taking beats to step back and step back in, don't stop talking to the other person. Just make sure that person is actually there when you're talking to them because . . . it's easy to win an argument in your head when you're writing your opponent's script.

This ever happen to you? You get in an argument with someone and you just fucking DESTROY them. You're like the DA at the end of a *Law & Order* episode questioning the teary-eyed suspect in court: *You don't just win the argument, you fucking crush them*. Yeah, that's never happened to me, either.

But how about this: Did you ever have an argument like that with someone . . . *in your head?* That's a trap I call "emotional shadowboxing." Any time you fight an imaginary argument with someone, or fantasize about delivering that perfect, blistering *Fuck you!* speech to them, you're emotional shadowboxing. All this does is reinforce what you already believe to be true: You're finding ways to justify and shore up whatever anger, frustration, or other negativity you're feeling, instead of easing it. In psychology we call this "confirmation bias." In Dr. V's office we call this "Shit I see every Tuesday." Even if you feel you lost the opportunity to say something you really needed to, the opportunity will present itself again when you're ready. You can even *make* it present itself, as long as you remember that being the Boss doesn't always mean being right.

When you're in an argument with someone, do you care about being "right"? Do you need to "win" the fight? If you're "right," does that mean you're "good"? Does that make the person you're in conflict with "bad"? Here's another question: *When was the last time being "right" in an argument got you anything?* I've thoroughly checked all written records of human history, and there is not one instance of someone getting laid because they knew they were "right." And unless a conflict is rooted in abuse or other toxic dysfunction, *"wrong" and "right" aren't available as sides to take.* Needing to be right lathers on a layer of blame to the other side, and when we blame, we surrender both our responsibility and our power. Give up the need to be right, and you're instantly the smartest person in the room. A Boss knows that conflict is a collision of needs, not a battle between good and evil. Which is why it's on you as the Boss to *negotiate a resolution to your conflict*. And I don't mean any of that *Art of the Deal* or *48 Laws of Power* bullshit. I'm talking about *real* negotiation, based in empathy.

Good Negotiation Begins Where You Want It to End

When you're the Boss, you don't wait for permission to find empathy, either for yourself or for the person you're in conflict with. Part of wisdom is being able to connect in conflict. When you can trust yourself to be objective (meaning that your answer to the question "Why did he do/say that?" isn't "Because he's an asshole!") ask yourself: *What does the person I'm in conflict with need that they're not getting? What's stopping them from getting it? How is this making them feel?* You don't have to blot out your own pain to recognize the reality of someone else's. Being able to find empathy for someone you're in conflict with lets you reframe the situation: It's still true that this person helped you feel bad. But did they really *want* to hurt you, or did they fuck up while trying to meet a need? This doesn't excuse the hurt done to you, but it can help you understand *why* it happened.

You won't be able to negotiate like a Boss *until* you find empathy. To find empathy, you have to compartmentalize your emotions enough to appreciate how your conflict looks from the opposite side. The person you're in conflict with isn't getting what they need either. Knowing that *you* want to help them get what they need sets the stage for cooperation instead of confrontation. A Boss opens a negotiation with, *"Tell me what you need, because I want to give it to you."*

There's a cliché that the sign of a good compromise is when both sides walk away disappointed. I wouldn't go so far as to call that #BadAdvice, but it's definitely #BummerAdvice. The real sign of a good compromise is when both sides walk away *satisfied*. "Satisfied" doesn't mean you got everything you wanted; it means you got all that you *needed*. When you're negotiating a conflict, you usually have to give up something (or things) that you want in order to get what you need.

Sorting your needs and wants isn't always simple, but you can start by answering this question: *Is the pain of staying in this conflict worse than the pain of giving up or going without whatever want is in question?* If the answer's "no," that's okay. It's why someone invented the term *nonnegotiable*. Some shit you just can't back down from. But if the answer is "yes," it's time for another Boss Move: *Be the first one to offer to give something up*.

Here's what I mean: It bothered my client Stephanie that her boyfriend Josh regularly "liked" photos of other women on Instagram. Josh's response was that of a Boss: "I had no idea you felt like that. I'm not lusting after these women, I'm just scrolling through Instagram 'liking' pics. I don't want to make you feel that way, so I'll stop doing it." Maybe that wouldn't work for every couple, but it worked for them. Stephanie's well-being and having peace in their relationship meant more to Josh than Instagram likes. (Again, not true for everyone.) Josh is a Boss because he was ready to be the first to give something up.

You don't need permission to negotiate, but you *do* need to be sure of what everyone's needs are. Don't try to make reality fit your assumptions. Talk to the person on the other side of the conflict, and *assure them that you want them to feel satisfied with how this conflict is resolved*. When the feeling is mutual, you'll know you're dealing with a fellow Boss and it'll be time to start negotiating. Empathetic, cooperative negotiation is a *reverse-engineering* project. Find that happy medium where you can give something up but still feel satisfied. Once you're there, work backwards, taking it step by step, piece by piece. Once you've done this, you'll have already cut the path forward.

And by the way, what you want, what you need, and what you're willing to give up can change in this process. That's okay. Negotiation is a process of change. A lot can shift in the space between a conflict's beginning and its resolution. This can happen within you, the other person, your relationship with each other, the conflict itself, or even the resolution. Conflict is one of the greatest change agents for a relationship there is, and often for the better. The best friends aren't made in good times; they're made in the conflicts they resolve together. But one thing remains unchanged throughout this whole process: *You remain a Boss.*

Earlier I mentioned conflicts rooted in abuse or other toxic behavior as an exception to using negotiation as a tool of resolution. But you still need to resolve toxic conflict if it creeps into your life, even if not through negotiation. If the only way someone thinks meeting a need happens is through hurting you in any way . . . that's a nonnegotiable conflict. But "nonnegotiable" doesn't mean unresolvable. Your answer to toxic, nonnegotiable conflicts is the same answer any Boss would have for a toxic employee unwilling to compromise: GTFO (which means "Get the Fuck Out," for everyone my age and older). Leave the job, the friendship, the relationship—whatever the situation is—and *stay away*. You *never* have to ask permission to escape abuse. And no one ever has permission to abuse you. Ever. A Boss takes no shit.

Forgiveness: One of the Most Self-Fulfilling Selfless Actions We Can Take

Whether you resolve your conflict through negotiating or by making an exit, one crucial step remains. And this is some #GoodAdvice you *do* need permission for—your own. *Give yourself permission to forgive yourself and who you were in conflict with.* Forgiveness doesn't mean accepting what you're forgiving, or that you're somehow sending a message that "everything's okay." Forgiveness isn't a denial of what you're forgiving; it's proof of your commitment to heal from it. Forgiveness redirects your energy from picking at a wound to healing it.

This might sound like New Age Hippie Bullshit until you look at the science on forgiveness. Scientific data link forgiveness with measurable improvements in physical, mental, and emotional health. So there is more in forgiveness for you than for the person you're forgiving. Forgiveness is a Boss Move in and of itself, but it's also the *result* of a series of Boss Moves.

The #BadAdvice of *Nobody Can Make You Feel Bad Without Your Permission* can't share the same space with forgiveness, because the two carry opposing emotional charges. Forgiveness can happen only after you recognize you've been hurt. *Nobody Can Make You Feel Bad Without Your Permission* denies that you even have something to forgive. And look, I know it may take awhile. It may even take a looooong while before you're ready to forgive the person you're in conflict with. That's okay. Just know that one day, you *will* be ready. Put a stickie note on this page so when that day comes, you can come back here if your forgiveness needs a jumpstart (because a Boss also knows when to ask for help).

Letting go, like feeling bad, is an emotional process. So you don't need anyone's permission (including your own) to do it. But you *can* decide to invite that feeling of letting go into your life. If you consistently practice empathy, express yourself, and connect with and confide in people you trust . . . *eventually you'll begin to let go*. When that feeling of letting go (aka "healing") eclipses the hurt, you're ready to forgive.

That leaves one last thing for you to do. *Tell whoever hurt you that you forgive them*. You need to actually say, *"I forgive you"*—out loud. Even if you've completely cut ties with the person you're forgiving, do this in a solitary moment. Saying something out loud helps make it real. It's the emotional equivalent of signing on the dotted line. As a Boss, you're the one responsible for making important shit like this official.

And yet, for as shitty as people can help you feel sometimes, it's also true that nobody needs your permission to help you feel good, either. So when someone's done something to hurt or piss you off and you feel overwhelmed, reach out to the people you can trust to help you feel better. Being the Boss doesn't mean you shoulder everything on your own. Let yourself be supported. Express how you feel. Dedicate yourself to the action of forgiveness, and eventually you'll start to let go. You won't even make a Boss Decision to let go. *You just will*.

A Boss Keeps Their Shit in Order

Bosses keep their shit in order. You can't leave crap lying out all over the office. The same holds true for your Head Office (see what I did there?). All that painful negativity cluttering up your headspace *has got to go*. You have to express that shit. A lot of people think the best way to do this is to write a letter to the person who hurt them with no intention of sending it. But here's the thing: *Writing a letter like this is just a kind of emotional shadowboxing*. You're having a conversation with this person in your head (actually, on paper).

The difference is your intention: You write a letter like this to express how you feel, not to "win" the conflict or otherwise try to feel "right." Keep your focus on your emotions. Assigning victim and villain roles or engaging in any other blame-related bullshit will not help. You can keep your process centered on you by writing more than one letter: Write a letter dedicated to each emotion that the conflict brought out. You can even go Martha Stewart on this shit by color coding your feelings, using matching paper for the letters connected to them.

Keeping the focus on your emotions also reality-tests your perceptions. In my own experience, I've found that nothing from my never-meant-to-send letters ever came up in actual conversations with the person I wrote them to. My emotions were real, but they were mine to engage and resolve. They had jack shit to do with reverse-engineering a solution to the conflict that inspired them. Expressing your feelings clears space in your Head Office to bring in the negotiating table.

Your Life Is an Exclusive, Limited-Run, One-Time-Only Engagement and You Have the Only Ticket: Because You're the Boss

Nobody Can Make You Feel Bad Without Your Permission tries to pass itself off as empowering, but it's really a bait-and-switch scheme. You're conned into thinking you have power when you're powerless, that you can control how other people affect your feelings, and that conflict is something you can choose to avoid through denial. You're also conned out of knowing yourself for who you really are. You're someone with the brains, grit, and creativity to see past the fear and pain a conflict can bring. Without denying the reality of how you feel, you can still find empathy for and understand someone who hurt you. Because of that, you're able to connect with the potential for opportunity and growth in a conflict. And I know this is all true because I know that *who you really are is a fucking Boss*. And just what are you the Boss of? YOU.

Your body, your mind, and your emotions are all components of a staggeringly complex system that works exclusively for you. It's a system designed to do one thing: *Create the life you want to live*. What does it mean to be the Boss of You? You are the Boss of every decision you will ever face. You are the Boss of your destiny. You are the Boss of your life-time. You always will be, and you always have been. You were born a Boss.

YOU WERE BORN A BOSS
#GOODADVICE

6

HONESTY IS THE BEST POLICY

Really? With this shit? Can you read it through your Valencia filter and fake news feed? If you're a human being, it's a given that you've been lied to and that you've lied to people. The same goes for me and every other person who has ever walked the Earth. *Honesty Is the Best Policy* is #BadAdvice. It's preachy. It's judgy. *It's dishonest*, because the world is full of deception.

In the few seconds that passed since you began reading this chapter, the following lies were told: A kid in Zurich told his mom he didn't eat the candy bar he just ate. A data systems analyst in Santa Monica told a homeless dude she didn't have any spare change. A man in Mumbai padded his résumé with bullshit. A woman in Boston just said she came. If those examples I-totally-did-not-make-up-on-the-spot-just-now didn't convince you, I have something else that will . . . *science, bit-chez*!!

A study from the 1970s suggested that the average person lies around two hundred times a day. But that was the seventies, so everyone was coked up and talking shit at the disco. We don't lie that much in the twenty-first century, right? Wrong. Recent data show people lie once every ten minutes in conversation with each other. Other research has found that when we're chatting online, we lie an average of every fifteen minutes. (It must take longer to type out bullshit.) The data vary, but they don't lie: *We do.*

So if everyone's lying so much, why isn't *Honesty Is the Best Policy* the #GoodAdvice everyone should heed? Because lying isn't a defect in human nature. Lying *is* nature. Lying is an act of deception, and deception is an evolutionary response to life-or-death situations. And when it comes to deception, humans are not a solo act.

It's Truth AND Deception That Hold Us Together

To either eat or avoid being eaten, animals play dead, pretend to be injured, pretend to be more or less dangerous than they really are, or try to make themselves appear a different size. When a butterfly's wings work together to create an illusion of a "false face" to confuse a predator, you don't call the butterfly a dirty fucking liar. It's a beautiful butterfly! You snap a pic and Instagram that shit (#ButterfliesOfInstagram). When the mimic octopus changes its shape and color to look like a deadly sea snake, we all say *Oooooo!*, not *Fuck you, you fucking phony!* Gorillas, fish, birds, even orchids engage in deception. Remember Koko, the famous gorilla who learned sign language? And remember how Koko cared for a kitten like it was her own baby? Koko once used sign language to blame that kitten for ripping a sink out of the wall. Koko was a brilliant ape, but she was a poor liar and a questionable parent. But why does Koko's deception seem shitty compared with those other examples? *Because deception is a valid response to mortal peril, but it's not valid for covering your ass.*

The same is true for us. Only a monster or a moron would think *Honesty Is the Best Policy* when the Nazis asked where the Jews were hiding. And only an asshole or an idiot would tell Grandma the true fate of that fugly holiday sweater she sent. Honesty is *not* the best policy when you're relying on deception to keep things from falling apart.

Deception Is Either a Symptom of Conspiracy or a Sign of Cooperation

Human civilization would crumble if no one lied about anything ever. We use deception to protect social bonds, and social bonds are how we survive and thrive. Social bonds enable cooperation—that fabulous thing we do that enabled us to build the pyramids, go to the moon, and share Postmates discount codes with each other. Dr. David Livingstone Smith, author of *Why We Lie: The Evolutionary Roots of Deception and the Unconscious Mind* (2004), commented to me: "The message that it's wrong to lie is frankly ridiculous. We kind of use our moral values, whatever they are, to try and make a call between what are the 'good' kind of lies and the 'bad' kind of lies. It gets very confusing, though, when this mythology is put around that lying is *just wrong*."

So when is honesty not the best policy? When is lying the right thing to do? Answer: *When a lie or hiding the truth will help an innocent.* It's why you compliment the horrible-but-homemade cookies your co-worker brings to the holiday party. It's why everyone claps for a kid barely scratching out "Mary Had a Little Lamb" on the violin. Need higher stakes? How about World War III? During the Cuban Missile Crisis, President John F. Kennedy deceived the public into believing he was taking a hard line against the Soviets. But in reality, he orchestrated secret cooperative meetings that stopped a nuclear war. This was kept secret from a lot of people at the top, including the vice president. (Insert stock footage of nuclear explosion.) Still think *Honesty Is the Best Policy*?

At the same time, we're stuck in a bizarre cultural moment. You know what I mean: *Alternative Facts. Fake News.* How can you expect to navigate between honesty and deception if you're conditioned to *always* accept and expect lies? In an attempt to adapt to the new (ab)normal, we've widened the avenue of acceptable and expected lying. What you *want* to be real matters more than what *is* real. Malignant deception has gone viral, and fraud is the new black. Instead of climbing out of the sewer, we're trying to get used to the smell. But lucky for us, we'll never get used to that stench. And it's not because *Honesty Is the Best Policy*. Because while we have a biological instinct to deceive, we have a biological aversion to lying when it hurts someone.

We're Designed to Lie for Each Other, Not to Each Other

Data suggest that your brain already knows when you should and shouldn't be lying. Your amygdala is a primitive part of your brain that processes and responds to fear. Researchers found that when people lied for their own benefit, their amygdala lit up: The act of lying made them afraid. But when the same people lied for the benefit of someone else, and there was nothing in it for them, their amygdala did not exhibit the same fear response.

Evolution has programmed your amygdala to make unethical, dishonest behavior feel bad. Your biology recognizes what the #BadAdvice of *Honesty Is the Best Policy* misses: The benefits of human connection and relationships are worth lying to protect.

We Lie Because Sometimes Trust Is Worth More Than the Truth

From the moment you entered the world, you began establishing trust, connecting and bonding with the people around you. Within hours of being born, an infant will orient her head to look into the eyes of whoever might be holding her. Soon after she'll turn her head toward her mom's voice, and finally, she'll start mimicking the facial expressions she sees on her caregivers' faces. Trust is a basic human need. It's the primary medium and currency of human connection. People can't function without trust, and quite often that trust is between strangers. How many times have you completely and unconditionally trusted someone, even when your life is on the line? Make that *especially* when your life is on the line. There's a general assumption that someone in a pilot's uniform or surgical scrubs isn't going to lie to you when it comes to your welfare. It seems like a huge leap of faith when you think about it, which is probably why you don't have to think about it: Trust is partly a function of your biology.

But so is deception. So you, along with the rest of humanity, are born with two powerful, conflicting instincts: the instinct to trust and the instinct to lie. It's such a powerful conflict that some scientists think we evolved a specific adaptation to deal with it. Dr. Timothy R. Levine's Truth Default Theory suggests that the potential benefits which come from trusting people throughout your life are so great that they are worth the risk of betrayal. Without trust, you wouldn't have access to friendship, fuck buddies, or the fruits of civilization. Which is why you need to nurture and protect the trust you share with others—even if you have to occasionally defend it with bullshit. Okay, so we agree: Honesty is not the best policy. We're going to bullshit each other sometimes. The question is, how are we going to bullshit each other? And for that, I have some #GoodAdvice.

Be Benevolent, Not Basic #GOODADVICE

Bullshit remains one of my favorite swear words. It's not quite as versatile as *Fuck*, but it still pulls off double duty as a noun ("That's bullshit!") and a verb ("I am not bullshitting you!"). *Horseshit* can't do that shit. Nobody accuses anyone of "horseshitting." And unlike horseshit, "bullshit" is not truly animal in origin. It is a purely human creation, which explains its success and adaptability. One of the distant ancestors of "bull," the Old French word *bole*, means "deception, trick, scheming, intrigue." As *bole* evolved into *bullshit*, its meaning expanded to encompass the unique way humans engage with and express their deceptive instincts. Those instincts are strong. And when they come knocking, it's on you to decide whether your style of bullshit is Benevolent or Basic.

Benevolent Bullshit is when you lie or otherwise keep the truth from someone to protect them and the social bond between you. Like when your best girlfriend asks *Be honest, do I look fat?* or *Be honest, was it time to put the cat down?* or *Be honest, was this tattoo a mistake?* Your friend isn't coming to you to hear THE TRUTH; she's coming to you for *comfort*. She trusts she can be vulnerable with you, that you'll support her and won't be a judgy asshole or kick her when she's down. And because you're an empathetic, caring friend, you do the empathetic, caring thing. You lie. You lie because it's a situation where the truth won't change anything. You lie to help ease your friend's pain. You lie because it's what good friends do for each other. You lie because sometimes *trust* is worth more than the truth. You lie because *Honesty Is the Best Policy* is #BadAdvice. You lie because you're a Benevolent Bullshitter.

Things get sketchy when you move into *Basic Bullshit*. Whenever you needlessly bullshit yourself or other people to avoid the truth or consequences of a situation, you're a Basic Bullshitter. I realize "basic" is usually reserved to describe women in a negative way, but no more! Bullshit doesn't discriminate, and neither do I. Blatant Basic Bullshit is easy to spot because it tends to show up in the same places: crime, politics, Silicon Valley, etc. But Basic Bullshit is usually more insidious. For example, you've probably sent or received a text like this: *Hey! I'm soooooo sorry but I don't think I can make it. Slammed at work all day and I'm exhausted. Ugh . . . I suck. Sorry!:(*

Maybe the part about being slammed at work is bullshit, but that's not the insidious part. Check out that *"I suck"* at the end. Is that there because you *really* think you suck? Or is it there because you don't want to hear *"You suck!"* because you flaked? That's called *false self-deprecation*. It's Basic Bullshit because you're trying to avoid the consequence of something *before you do it*. It's always a dick move to fuck someone over and try to get away with it ahead of time.

Another Basic Bullshit move is to say "I'm just being honest" when what you really mean is "I'm just being cruel." Total Basic Bullshit. How many times have you seen someone use "just being honest" as a cover for cruelty? (Mindfuck Alert: Using "Being Honest" as a cover for *anything* is not being honest.) That person's not keep'n it real; they're being a real asshole. It's even possible for you to Basic Bullshit someone without realizing it.

Deception May Be Universal, But Only Human Beings Bullshit

Can you remember the last time you blinked? Probably not, because it's an involuntary reflex. Do you remember the last time you bullshitted? You might not, because sometimes your reflex response to a situation is to bullshit. The research showing that people lie every ten minutes came from a study led by Dr. Robert Feldman. (No relation to my co-writer Paul Feldman's Uncle Bob, aka Dr. Robert Feldman, a retired urologist who lives in Great Neck, New York; but then again, Paul could be lying.) So what were Feldman's Basic Bullshitters lying about? Themselves. Feldman believes that the Basic Bullshit he observed was tied to self-esteem. When his subjects felt their self-esteem or self-image threatened, they didn't just lie, they lied without realizing it.

And here's where it gets really weird: The reflex for deception is rooted in your amygdala, the part of your brain that feels threatened by a self-serving lie. As far as your amygdala's concerned, you're still an Ice Age cave-dweller who could be a breath away from becoming lunch for a saber-toothed cat. A threat to your self-image is perceived as an actual threat to your *physical self*, because your amygdala frames *any* threatening situation as IMPENDING FUCKING DOOM. That primal animal fear provokes a primal animal response of defensive deception, which can lead to Basic Bullshitting.

So are Feldman's lie-every-ten-minutes subjects any different from the mimic octopus's sea snake impression? Yes. Feldman elaborated on this when we discussed his research: "There's a lot of evidence that different species use deception as a means for getting along in the world. But I think it's really important to keep in mind that we also learn to lie. We're taught to lie. We use it as a social tactic. And it's a very effective one. I don't think it's driven *totally* by evolutionary, genetic, or social factors; I think it's a combination of the three." It is true that you have an instinct to bullshit your way out of a threatening situation. But you have more working for you than instinct. You have intelligence. You have intuition. You can learn to outsmart Basic Bullshit.

Life Is Too Short to Eat Bad Food, Miss Too Many Sunsets, or Waste Time with Basic Bullshittery

Outsmarting Basic Bullshit starts with getting yourself *unused* to it. Remember that data about your brain's amygdala responding with fear when you lie? The same study found that consistently lying for your own benefit (Basic Bullshitting) reduces the amygdala's response. The researchers called this a "blunted response." Put another way, the data show that Basic Bullshitting on the regs hits the mute button on your conscience. If you'd rather mute your Basic Bullshit, you'll need to sharpen that blunted response.

This means answering some tough questions: *Who is on the receiving end of most of your Basic Bullshit? The people you work with? Your friends? Your family? The person you're fucking and/or want to fuck? Someone you've just met?* If you're not sure where to start looking, start with any and all of your bullshit excuses. Don't say you got stuck in traffic when you really got stuck binge-watching *Marriage Boot Camp*. Don't add inches or subtract pounds (unless you're using photo editor on Insta). And for fuck's sake, don't say you came when you didn't. Develop awareness around your Basic Bullshit, and it will become less and less of a thoughtless reflex.

And just like giving up refined sugar, there are legitimate health benefits to reducing and staying aware of your Basic Bullshit. Psychology professor Anita Kelly asked a group of study participants to make a conscious effort not to lie over a period of ten weeks. At the end of the ten weeks, Kelly's subjects reported feeling less sadness and stress along with having fewer headaches and fewer sore throats. They also thought that the quality of their relationships had improved.

But even after you clean up the Basic Bullshit in your relationships, what about when *you're* the target of your Basic Bullshit? How can you decide to stop bullshitting yourself *if you don't know you're bullshitting yourself*?

You Can't Put Basic Bullshit Behind You Until You Face It Up Front

Denial, aka "Lying to Yourself," is a form of bullshit that can be either Benevolent or Basic. Benevolent Denial can help people deal with hardships and trauma. But it's supposed to wear off after a while, allowing for a process where you gradually surrender your denial in exchange for acceptance. For example, if you're nervous about giving a speech and you "psych yourself up" to overcome the fear, you're denying your anxiety by bullshitting yourself into confidence. If the deception ends there, it's Benevolent Bullshit. Which is good. But what if your denial doesn't wear off? When you *consistently* bullshit yourself to avoid a truth, you're stuck in denial and rolling deep in Basic Bullshit. Which is bad. But what if you're *stuck* in Basic Denial? What are the symptoms you need to watch for?

Think about the last few times you've fucked up. Did you accept responsibility, or did you try to minimize, justify, or blame away your fuckup? Did you recognize the cause and effect you created, or did you make that bullshit excuse of *It Just Happened!* In your everyday life, do you reflect on how what you say and do affects people, or do you bullshit yourself into being an oblivious ass? And look, don't get too wound up worrying about whether you're a chronic Basic Bullshitter: You'd be a raging psychopath with no interest in this book if you were. Instead, watch for any singular moments that remind you of the situations I just described. This might involve some emotional heavy lifting for you, so it's okay if it takes some time to find these answers.

You can start this process by having a conversation with someone you trust, or even with yourself. (Don't laugh; that can really work.) Or you can write out your questions and answers on paper. Don't be afraid to dig through your own bullshit, and whatever bullshit you've laid on other people. It counts for a lot. You're confronting your own denial. A better understanding of the nuance between Basic Bullshit and Benevolent Bullshit leads to a better understanding of your own humanity—something you will *never* get from this chapter's #BadAdvice of *Honesty Is the Best Policy*.

Right now you're probably operating on a bullshit surplus, and you want to change that (I hope). But before you can change yourself, you have to forgive yourself. Do it. Grant yourself a one-time-only Blanket Bullshit Amnesty. Reflect on every time you've Basic Bullshitted either you or someone else—and then forgive yourself. Forgive yourself for any and all of your Basic Bullshit. Instead of judging your behavior as "bad" because it didn't measure up to the impossible standard of *Honesty Is the Best Policy*, try to perceive it as imperfect *human* behavior. Human behavior can transcend its imperfection and messiness, because it's also changeable—but only after forgiveness. Forgiveness opens the way for acceptance, and acceptance opens the way for change. And that's no bullshit.

There's a Stronger You Waiting on the Other Side of Pain

Unfortunately, eliminating your own Basic Bullshit doesn't protect you from someone else's. Since it's in your DNA to trust people, you're also preprogrammed to risk being betrayed. This is the shitty side of the trust equation, because betrayal fucking sucks. Stephen King wrote that fear begins when the "good fabric of things" begins to unravel with "shocking suddenness." The feeling of betrayal begins in a similar way. Betrayal is the feeling that accompanies the discovery that you've been bullshitted. Your reality feels violated.

The reason betrayal can be so devastating is because it is a breed of grief. You're mourning a loss of trust, closeness, and security. You mourn the loss of who you *thought* someone was. Your body gets hit as hard as your heart and mind. Betrayal shakes up your parasympathetic nervous system, which regulates your appetite, sleep, and respiration. You start looking like a walking list of side effects from a drug commercial: insomnia, loss of appetite, shortness of breath. It's easy to spiral down and feel even shittier because on top of dealing with betrayal, your physical needs aren't being met. Meanwhile, in your brain's basement, your sweaty, paranoid amygdala perceives betrayal as a threat: The Fight, Flight, or Freeze response skews your perception even more.

Betrayal is one of the most thorough fuck-overs you can experience. The excruciating feeling of betrayal is another reason why the #BadAdvice of *Honesty Is the Best Policy* seems comforting. Most of us are trusting people who want to trust and be trusted. So if everyone would just follow this #BadAdvice, no one will ever have to feel betrayed. But that's not reality. You can't bullshit your way out of feeling betrayed. But don't confuse being in pain with being powerless, because even though betrayal can change who you are, it doesn't change you permanently.

No Matter How Good or Bad a Single Day Is, You Will Outlast It

Emotions come and go. Whether it's through writing, another medium, or even just talking to someone else about how you feel, exploring and expressing your feelings of betrayal helps you accept those feelings and empowers you. By accepting and expressing feelings, you give yourself the power and permission to change them. Still, part of your recovery from betrayal happens in the same way physical healing does: Your mind and body know how to repair themselves without you doing anything. Give them time. Take care of yourself. Do something that gets you moving, which can help you focus on something else, especially if you're not alone when you do it. And if you've recently been betrayed, or reading this is bringing up the pain of a past betrayal, I want you to know that it's *never* wrong to trust. It's *never* wrong to love.

Your instinct to trust is betrayal-proof, and you need to remind yourself of that. Surround yourself with people you trust, like, and admire—people who carry a "positive charge." Create a consistent and positive social experience for yourself, even when you're feeling less than positive. Spending time with people to whom you feel close can soothe the hurt of betrayal and remind you of your ability to trust. It's not like you have a choice anyway. As a social animal living in a complex, interconnected society, you are going to keep on trusting. You need to, and you will. It's part of your biological programming. As much as we seem hardwired to bullshit, we're *harderwired* to trust.

Human Connection: The Original World Wide Web

Honesty Is the Best Policy denies this truth about trust, and it denies the inevitability of bullshit. It's a given that you will both bullshit and be bullshitted. And that's not because you're a rotten liar living in a rotten, liar-infested world. You are one of billions of unique, sensitive, courageous, and beautiful creatures, desperately trying to make sense of this daz-

zling mess called life. In doing so, you're carrying on one of
the oldest human traditions. It's also what inspired people to
turn to #BadAdvice in the first place, because being human
is a tough fucking job. It's messy. It's confusing. It's painful.
But it's also exciting. It's joyous. It's beautiful.

Honesty is the Best Policy is #BadAdvice because it reduces
the complex, multifaceted experience of life into something
that is oversimplified, binary, and absolute. Life is none of
those things, and neither are you. You were born into an
ongoing conflict between your protective instinct to deceive
and your connective instinct to trust: *And it can be fucking
hard to navigate their influences.* Learning to discern Benevolent Bullshit from Basic Bullshit eases your learning curve
toward understanding your own deceptive instinct. Choosing to be a Benevolent Bullshitter helps you create and sustain genuine connections with people. You remake yourself
as someone who strives to bullshit only when bullshitting
protects a social bond or the trust that sustains that bond.

Because of this, you're able to trust better and more
courageously. Not because you're immune to betrayal; only
#BadAdvice promises to eliminate the potential for pain.
You trust with courage because you understand that the re-
wards of trust are worth the risk of betrayal. Every connection you make opens another potential avenue for goodness
and opportunity to enter your life. That's something you will
have created for yourself. It won't happen because you took
the #BadAdvice of *Honesty Is the Best Policy*, but because
you were able to reach a more honest understanding of the

strength and flaw you and I share with everyone else: a trusting heart. With that understanding and strength comes your responsibility to yourself to be benevolent, not basic.

BE BENEVOLENT, NOT BASIC
#GOODADVICE

7

FOLLOW YOUR BLISS

No one in the history of humankind has ever blissfully followed their way into success and fulfillment. I can be certain of this because I checked with one of those nice docents at the Museum of Natural History. *Follow Your Bliss* is the #BadAdvice offered when you wonder *What do I want to do with my life?*, usually in reference to a career or profession. It's a question you might ponder a lot, because it's something you're constantly being asked, usually in the form of *What do you do?* Well . . . you *do* a lot of things. Your job is one of them, but it's not the sum total of your identity as a human being. *Follow Your Bliss* is #BadAdvice because it tricks you into believing that pleasure is the same thing as fulfillment. It isn't: This #BadAdvice is also #StupidAdvice.

The first word of this #BadAdvice is #Annoying just on

its own: *Follow*. Do you really want one of your life's main directives to be *following* something? The word "follow" and its variations "following" and "followers" are not the calling cards of greatness. *She followed him over the edge. He duped his following out of millions. How many online followers do you have?* It's a word mostly associated with mindlessness or nothingness. And what is *Bliss*? A state of ongoing, near-catatonic happiness? Where are they hiring for that?

The answer to *What do you do?* is bigger than your career, because it's *everything* you do—what you say, what you think, how you act, who you love—all of it. But that's not what you're taught. You're deceived into believing that your job *is all you are*. And that's just not true. Alain de Botton, author of *Status Anxiety* (2004), observed that hundreds of years ago, your identity had less to do with your job and more to do with who your family was and where you came from (which is just as fucked-up). But now, de Botton says, our identities are fused with our jobs. In other words, we live in a culture that blindly and mercilessly assumes that what you do, specifically, *what you get paid to do*, is who you *are*. If your job isn't impressive, neither are you. You're a *loser*. De Botton also points out that the modern context we have for the word "loser," meaning someone who's a failure, is relatively recent. He notes that in medieval times, people struggling or at the bottom of society were called "unfortunates." Today they're called "losers." The difference? A loser is at fault for being a loser. So when your day job doesn't match your dream job, being asked *What do you do?* can be a terrifying question: *You're about to be ex-*

posed as a worthless piece of shit loser! So you do what any worthless piece of shit loser desperate for answers does: You Google that shit.

Google

what should I do
_____
what should I do
what should I do **with my life**

You read life-hack blogs, list articles, maybe visit the websites of a few self-appointed experts, each claiming to have the Answer to Everything. Maybe you talk to a few friends you think are smarter than you, because *they* might know what you want to do with your life. Somewhere in your searching, you will inevitably hear *Follow Your Bliss*, or one of its variations. *Follow Your Bliss. Follow Your Dream. Do What You Love, and You'll Never Work Another Day in Your Life.* Like the Law of Attraction and other self-help fairy tales, *Follow Your Bliss* disguises consumerism as spirituality: *If you get everything you want, you'll always be happy.* That is some fuck'n #BadAdvice. But get this. In its *original* form, *Follow Your Bliss* was actually #AwesomeAdvice from a brilliant man.

Your Life Is the Story Where You Choose to Be the Hero

Joseph Campbell was a world-renowned scholar and professor of literature who is best known for his work in mythology and comparative religions. His work revealed, among other things, how the myths and folk stories of all cultures share common elements. These elements reflect deeper truths about human nature, universal emotional needs, and the basic experience of being alive. Campbell elaborated on the meaning of *Follow Your Bliss* in his collaboration with Bill Moyers, *The Power of Myth*: "Follow your bliss and don't be afraid, and doors will open where you didn't know they were going to be." Campbell defined "following your bliss" as keeping your mind "on those moments when you feel most happy, when you really are happy—not excited, not just thrilled, but deeply happy."

He isn't talking about the way a job makes you feel; he means the way *life* makes you feel. *Follow Your Bliss* is a poignant insight into the human condition that's been reduced to career advice. It implies that when you turn Having Fun into Going to Work, you win at life. Even Campbell saw the meaning in his words get lost. When his students started using "Follow Your Bliss" as a license to get wasted all the time, he supposedly said, "I should have said 'Follow Your Blisters.'"

Bliss isn't eternal happiness or a perpetually satisfied pleasure center. It's how you feel when you find meaning and purpose in life. "If you follow your bliss," Campbell said, "you put yourself on a kind of track that has been there all the while, waiting for you, and the life that you ought to be living is the one you are living. Wherever you are—if you are following your bliss, you are enjoying that refreshment, that life within you, all the time." I believe the doors Campbell said would open are doors to a deeper understanding and appreciation of life and your place in the world. They're a gateway to an ongoing path, not the dead end of some perfect and imaginary achievement. Campbell fed society wisdom, and society spat it back as #BadAdvice.

Money Is Powerful, but It's Not the Only Power You Can Access

Watering down Joseph Campbell's thoughts on the Meaning of Life to a job fair cliché could happen only in the comfort of the First World, where dogs are prescribed Prozac. The #BadAdvice of *Follow Your Bliss* fails again here because it assumes that if you find a fun and/or impressive way to meet your basic needs (aka a "cool job"), you'll be a "success." What the fuck does *that* even mean? It fails because this #BadAdvice carries a twisted assumption that when you *Follow Your Bliss*, truckloads of cash aren't far behind. It's also implied in similar sayings such as *Do what you love and the money will follow.* That can be true, but it's certainly not *always* true. And even if it were, a good amount of scientific data suggest that money *can't* buy happiness.

Studies reveal that people's reported feelings of happiness increase with their income, only *up until their cost of living is covered*. After that, getting more money doesn't move the needle. Money can *help* bring happiness because it can help create stability, but finding stability doesn't mean you've found fulfillment. Research shows that *how* you work can possibly be even more important than *what* your work is. Psychologist Barry Schwartz believes that before factories arrived on the scene, the work most people did differed every day. Each day called for new problem-solving skills, creativity, and ingenuity. This ultimately led to fulfillment, meaning, and purpose. Factory work ended that. Each worker did the same assigned job all day, every day. Fulfillment, meaning, and purpose in daily life vanished.

Reducing compensation to only a paycheck also reduces *you*. It reduces your meaning and purpose in life to survival, nothing more. I'm not saying material success and comfort don't matter, only that they matter *to a point*. My client Lydia was a high-powered, wealthy attorney. She was driven, determined, and amazing at her job. She was also perpetually exhausted and unfulfilled and one of the most miserable people I'd ever met. Most of our discussions revolved around how unhappy her job made her. It polluted every other aspect of her life. Even with the corner office, the Bentley coupe, and the Bel Air zip code, she was still alone, lonely, and only surviving. Lydia sweated blood building a career that made her wealthy. But that career also left her exhausted, empty, and *blissless*. I know what you're thinking. *Oh, boo hoo. Lydia the rich-ass lawyer is sad. I sure hope her tears don't stain her Bentley's leather seats on her way to that champagne brunch.*

Yes, Lydia was a privileged person. But privilege doesn't

insulate anyone from feeling pain and having problems. *Money Can't Buy Happiness*: It's a scientific truth. But the multibillion-dollar advertising industry has a habit of drowning out both truth and science. It's dedicated to persuading you of the healing power of "retail therapy" (aka buying shit to make you feel happy). Which is also why we have no empathy for people who have stuff: *Having stuff is supposed to make everyone happy. They have stuff, so what the fuck's their problem?* At the same time, it helps explain our bizarre cultural resentment of the poor: *You're poor because you're lazy. Grab those bootstraps, make some money, and buy some stuff. Your suffering is a real downer. Jeez, some people are so self-absorbed.*

Trying to *Follow Your Bliss* is a never-ending search to find and possess that elusive magic *something* that will fulfill your every need. But success isn't having a shit ton of money and/or stuff. So if it's not bliss, just what the hell are we following?

The Human Race Is Not a Rat Race

In 1953, James Olds and Peter Milner wired up a rat so that the rat could stimulate a certain part of its brain by pushing a lever. Olds and Milner thought they had discovered the "bliss center" of the brain, because the rat kept hitting that lever, over and over again. The rat didn't care about eating, sleeping, or fucking. Walking over electrified metal didn't deter the rat: Charred paws were worth another hit from the lever. All that mattered was the next hit. Years later, when a similar experiment was carried out with humans, scientists found that it wasn't bliss the rat was experiencing. Instead, the people described feeling a kind of intense agitation and expectation. They felt they were on the verge of something really great happening. Every jolt they got kept them at that point of intense, yet still unfulfilled pleasure. *That* was the feeling both they and the rat were hooked on. The human subjects became just as addicted to dosing themselves with that jolt as the rat had been, giving themselves psychological blue balls. Instant Hell, at the touch of a button marked "Bliss."

Your brain is no different, and neither is mine. We are addicted to wanting to be happy. And where there's addiction, there are dealers. Which is why it's so easy to find yourself strung out on a never-ending bliss chase. Between advertising, social media, and our society's general addiction to either quick fixes or disposability, there's no shortage of false bliss buttons pushing themselves on you.

British philosopher Alan Watts eloquently described this process and its progress over your lifetime:

> *In nursery school, they say you are getting*
> *ready to go on to kindergarten. And then first*
> *grade is coming up and second grade and third*
> *grade. They say you are gradually climbing the*
> *ladder, making progress. [And then there's high*

*school and college] and you go out into the
business world with your suit and diploma. . . .
And then finally . . . you wake up one morning
as vice president of the firm, and you say to
yourself, "I've arrived. But I've been cheated.
Something is missing." [And then you retire],
thinking that this is the attainment of the goal
of life. . . . [But] you're a phantom. . . . You are
just nowhere, because you never were told,
and you never realized, that eternity is now.*

Watts is describing a lifetime of living like the rat in the experiment. It's a mentality described as "Wanting Mind" by Dr. Ronald Alexander, psychotherapist and the author of *Wise Mind, Open Mind: Finding Purpose and Meaning in Times of Crisis, Loss, and Change* (2009). I asked him to expand on this idea: "Everything in Western culture is geared toward [an idea] that if you succeed, if you aspire for more, have more, do more, you will eventually arrive at happiness and fulfillment. And that's a fantasy." Alexander connects the idea of Wanting Mind to a similar concept in Buddhism with an eerily accurate name: *hungry ghost*. "When you don't have what you want, you suffer. And then you discover when you arrive at getting what you want, *that* causes pain and suffering." Alexander explained why. "If your Self is primarily fixated [on the belief] that something from the external world is going to fill up an already inherent sense of emptiness, when you arrive at what you think is going to make you happy, you discover, 'Oh wow, that's not really going to touch into the core of my soul, or the core of my being, or in some way really repair or heal.'"

But you're not doomed to live your life as a hungry ghost. You don't have to settle for living like a rat forever waiting for the next hit off the Bliss Button. (This wouldn't be much of a self-help book if my premise was that life is an unending cycle of shit, pain, and despair from which death is the only escape.) The difference between the fulfillment of life and Wanting Mind isn't what you've done or what you have, but instead what Alexander calls your *contentment and happiness quotient*:

> *When you arrive at what you think will give you what you want, if you have a high quotient of happiness and contentment, then you'll be able to experience pleasure, joy, ambition, accomplishment, and achievement, and it will fill you up. Fulfillment, purpose, meaning, connection, and feeling that what you do and who you are matter help maintain your quotient of contentment and happiness.*

You can't buy any of what Alexander lists, even with an Amazon Prime membership. And you don't arrive at the meaningful fulfillment and satisfaction Campbell described by *following* anything. You don't arrive at bliss at all: *You create it.* But you don't create your bliss out of nothing. Bliss begins to manifest once you get a grip on a much more primal substance: *your grit.*

Grip Your Grit #GOODADVICE

Grip is a better start for a piece of advice than *Follow*. It's empowering. When you grip something, you know you have a firm hold on it *and* you understand it. One of humanity's greatest strengths comes from our *grip*. Anthropologists like to make a big deal of our opposable thumbs: They're what allowed us to make all our unique advancements in technology, science, and masturbation. I believe it was Charles Darwin who so famously wrote, *Hey, check out all this amazing shit only we can do because of our thumbs!* But the strength of our grip exceeds the physical realm. Human beings are meaning-seeking and meaning-making creatures. Psychologists theorize that this is rooted in a survival instinct. *Finding or creating meaning in life gives you a stronger grip on understanding yourself and the world around you.* This helps you to better adapt and thrive.

And since meaning is so important, just what the hell is *grit*? Grit is the armor that lets you take a punch when life throws one at you. Grit is the wisdom to value the responsibility of commitment over the desire for things to always be easy. Psychologist Angela Lee Duckworth has researched and written extensively on grit. She describes it as "passion and perseverance for very long-term goals. Grit is having stamina. Grit is sticking with your future, day in, day out, not just for the week, not just for the month, but for years, and working really hard to make that future a reality. Grit is living life like it's a marathon, not a sprint."

Grit is heroic. Grit is the vital ingredient of that beloved human phenomenon *The Triumph of the Underdog*. We're inspired by stories of grit. Stories about people who busted their ass and sweated blood to beat the odds to achieve something. *Rocky. Harry Potter. An Equally Well-Known Franchise Centered on a Nonwhite Female Character That Somebody Should Make.* We love these stories because they reflect what we all so desperately hope is within us: *grit.* I'm here to tell you: You don't have to hope for it. I promise you, *You have grit.* Grit and the heroism it creates are more accessible than you think.

Duckworth's research, which evaluated successful people ranging from West Point cadets to National Spelling Bee winners to top performers in the private sector, found that despite their varying backgrounds and ages, races, and talents, successful people all shared the unifying characteristic of grit. *Everyone* has grit. My grit went into the writing of this book, and your grit is why you're reading it.

I love the word "grit." (Thanks, Angela!) I love it because it sounds like what it is: a substance that's at once granular and indestructible. Something tough and earthy. Grit doesn't fit neatly into the world of modern self-helpy fads. It's not easy or fast. It's not even always pain free. Gritty people perceive success and failure not as singular moments, but as points on a continuum. Grit is trust in your own worth and ability, to the point of heroic stubbornness. It's the fuel that drives you to get back up after you've been knocked down. You don't expect everything to always be easy, because you know you can handle it when things get hard.

And yet, even with our amazing grip and the wonders of grit, human beings remain creatures who are prone to fuckups. Especially when we operate off unchallenged #BadAdvice. You might think you would be searching for and making meaning as you tried to *Follow Your Bliss*, but you'd be following an illusion that was leading you nowhere. That doesn't take grit: All you need for that is a rat paw and a Bliss Button. But look, I get it. The question of *How do I find meaning and purpose in life?* is just as heavy and impossible to answer as *What do you do?* And aren't you still fucked if you can't answer it? Not at all. In fact you don't even need to answer it, because to *Grip Your Grit*, you begin with answering a completely different question.

How Do You Want to Give Back in Life?

When you feel like what you do matters, and when what you do connects you to others in a meaningful way, you will love what you do. Ask yourself how you *want* to give back in life, and your focus will shift from what you want to take from the world to what you have to offer it. This doesn't mean it will always be fun or easy. It doesn't mean you won't sometimes feel stressed, frustrated, or exhausted. What you won't feel is bored, directionless, or without purpose. You'll have a grip on who you are and why you do what you do, because you'll have a *Grip on Your Grit*.

Workplace evidence backs this up, and it's probably not from the workplace you were expecting. Amy Wrzesniewski, a professor of organizational behavior, revealed the immense meaning the custodial staff at hospitals found in their work. One worker rearranged the artwork from room to room for comatose patients, in the hopes that having different art on the walls might help them somehow. Another janitor wanted to comfort a patient's father, so he mopped the patient's room twice—once to clean it, the second time to be *seen* cleaning it. Another worker risked getting in trouble and skipped vacuuming because she saw that an exhausted family was finally getting some sleep. There was no extra pay for this, no official recognition. These workers weren't looking for it, anyway. The genuine fulfillment and meaning they found in their work is what drove them. It was an affirmation that their work mattered, and by extension, *so did they*. In *Gripping Their Grit*, these people found fulfillment and meaning (in other words, *bliss*) in a job few would consider doing.

Maybe you won't decide on a career as a hospital janitor, but hopefully your perspective on what makes for "meaningful work" is just a little more open to the unexpected. My dad taught me this. He's been an auto mechanic for forty-five years, mostly at the same shop. He grew up in a working-class Italian neighborhood on the outskirts of Philadelphia, and I don't think anyone ever told him to Follow His Bliss. And I can tell you, he wouldn't strike you as the world's most blissful auto mechanic.

"Hey Dad, how ya do'n?"

"I worked all day. How was your day?"

I've asked him, more than once, "Don't you want to try something else?" His answer is always the same: "Why? I work with my buddies there, I love it." It isn't just being a mechanic that my dad loves, it's that the job makes him feel important, valued, and connected to other people. It's given him opportunities to learn, hone, and pass on a unique set of skills. Being a mechanic makes my dad feel like he matters, because he does. He's *Gripped His Grit*. Why would he leave that?

You will *Grip Your Grit* when you find something that you enjoy doing that provides connection with others and the sense that you are helping the world. You'll find passion for your work that you never would have found if you tried to *Follow Your Bliss*. As Mike Rowe, host of the reality show *Dirty Jobs*, so wisely said: "You don't follow your passion. You always bring it with you, but you never follow it."

What You Aspire to Be Is Already Within You

From both scientific and spiritual angles, an involuntary, outward-expanding energy is native to all living things. It's a biological reality. Seeds expand into trees. Eggs expand into birds. Humans expand, too. When was the last time you had to make sure your cells were dividing or that your lungs were properly exchanging the carbon dioxide in your blood with oxygen? And you do all this, and more, *even in your fucking sleep!* Your body has a built-in intelligence that enables you to perform all these biological miracles. And while you may not be aware of it yet, a similar built-in intelligence lies within you that already knows *Who You Are* and *What You Do.* You want those answers? Start asking questions.

Who are you? Are you a Light Bringer? A Truth Seeker? A Teacher? An Artist? A Storyteller? A Healer? A Builder? A Planner? An Advisor? A Caretaker? A Guardian? Are you a combination of some or all of these things, or others not listed?

If you don't know, that's okay. Skip to the next questions: *What would I do for nothing, but give anything to do? What's the thing I'd happily line up for eight hours in the rain to do? What do I always make time for? What makes me forget time? What would I do whether I get paid for it or not?* Whatever your answer (or answers) is, it *is* you. *What You Do* is not *Who You Are;* instead, *Who You Are* reveals *What You Do.* Once you know what that is, *figure out how to do it for other people.* In doing this, you forge a powerful connection, because you've created a way to find joy in being of service to others. And by the way, you can be of service in a professional context (in other words, *you can get paid for it*). Your shift in intention from selfish to selfless opens the way to *Grip Your Grit.*

When a woman named Samantha first came to see me,

she was surviving as a bank teller because she didn't yet know she was a Teacher. But during our talks about "what she wanted to do," it became clearer and clearer that Sam was a born Teacher. She began to recognize that throughout her life, she had found connection and meaning by passing on knowledge to others. Still, the idea of standing in front of a group of people, the way teachers often do, terrified her. So she had to get both curious and creative about how she answered the question "What does a teacher do?" She had to be open to widening her perceptions. So Samantha began a process of seeking and sampling that led her to the field of occupational therapy. She now works one-on-one, teaching babies and toddlers in a way that compensates her in heart, mind, soul—and wallet.

"Ready" Is a Place You Reach Only Through Commitment

Your *Grip on Grit* is only as strong as your commitment to it. How do you define commitment? *Can* you define commitment? Our society seems to have a contradictory understanding of it. One definition describes commitment as "the state or quality of being dedicated to a cause, activity, etc.," while another says that commitment is "an engagement or obligation that restricts freedom of action." This dual definition is part of the problem: Too many of us confuse being dedicated to something with being held back by whatever we're dedicated to. We view commitment as an inflexible state of being, as if commitment imprisons us. But the opposite is true. Real commitment is about flexibility and being able to adapt. In those moments when you are able to be flexible, commitment doesn't leave you feeling imprisoned, it leaves you feeling *motivated*. Commitment is part of what enables you to *Grip Your Grit*, because it helps create *motivation*.

Motivation: If You Can Create Just a Little, It Will Make More of Itself

A lot of people think that motivation is a character strength, but it's not. Motivation is an emotion. And like any other emotion, it ebbs and flows on your emotional tides. As an emotion, motivation is an involuntary response to a stimulus, not a state of being you decide to enter. What we're motivated to do varies from person to person, but everyone feels motivated in some way. So you will feel motivated no matter what. And although you can't make yourself feel instantly motivated, *you can help yourself feel that way*. You invite motivation into your life through the action of commitment. Even if you're not especially motivated to hit the gym, when you keep your commitment and drag your ass in, chances are you'll start feeling motivated once you're there. And then you'll be primed to forge commitment and motivation into another Grit-Gripping tool: *willpower*.

Willpower Is Being Able to Give Up What's in Front of You for What's Yet to Be Revealed Within You

People often talk about willpower as if it were some in-born virtue, something you either have or don't have. That's bullshit. Willpower is a psychological muscle, like critical thinking, a self-observing ego, and a well-cultivated sexual imagination. The more you exercise it, the stronger it gets. And you don't even need a commitment to exercise your will-power. Research suggests that something as simple as using your nondominant hand to brush your teeth or open a door can begin building and exercising your willpower. It creates a physical sensation of your ability to effect immediate, real change in yourself. Commitment, motivation, and willpower are essential to establishing and maintaining your *Grip on Your Grit*. But if you don't want to lose your grip, it better be adaptable.

Destiny Changes with the Direction You're Walking In

Adapting is not the same thing as *abandoning*. Trying differ-ent things and discovering what you don't like may be the only way to find out what you do like. Changing direction is part of the process. If something you thought would bring joy doesn't, then recommit to something else. Why wouldn't you? In his book *Time Enough for Love* (1973) the science fiction writer Robert Heinlein wrote "specialization is for insects." Meaning ants and bees might be specifically designed to do only one thing their whole lives, but *you* are a vessel of limitless potential.

The director of the tech innovation firm X (formerly Google X), Astro Teller, gives bonuses to employees who voluntarily end their failing projects because he understands that changing direction when something doesn't work isn't "failing." Failure is when you keep on going in the same direction knowing it's a dead end. Changing your mind isn't failing. Stopping one thing and starting another isn't failing. And by the way, you only really stop when you're dead. So if you're alive, you have no excuse . . . no matter how badly you might want one.

Life Is a Process of Movement and Change, Not Static Results

My friend Michael is now the CEO of a tremendously successful internet company. Which I never would have predicted when we met. When Michael and I were introduced, he was the top resident at the University of Maryland School of Medicine. The same creativity, curiosity, and drive that inspired Michael to work his way to top resident inspired him to change directions. The fact that he had completed medical school and was already teaching other medical students did not stop him. Michael left medicine entirely to start that booming company.

Some might have seen that decision as "failing" or "a big fucking mistake." But as my mom would say, I've got a news flash for ya: By making that change, he was living life to the fullest.

Michael didn't regret his time as a resident: It fed his fascination with biology, medicine, and science. He *Gripped His Grit* as a doctor, and he continued to *Grip His Grit* as an entrepreneur. The direction of Michael's commitment shifted, his profession changed, but his grit remained. Cultivating your grit does more than give you something to grip; it provides you with something to stay grounded in. What you choose to do may change, but your gritty approach remains constant.

Learning Only Stops with Your Heartbeat

Once you've figured out the particulars of how you'll *Grip Your Grit*, jump in, explore your field, and find out as much as you can. To make a profession of *Gripping Your Grit*, you can't half-ass it. *You have to kick ass—and want to do so.* Which means you need to hone your skills and abilities. Classes or professional training are great if they're an option, but formal instruction isn't always available for every field.

But perhaps even more important than classes and instruction is finding your *professional community*—the people already *Gripping Their Grit* in a way similar to you. You need to find what Angela Duckworth calls a *gritty mentor.* Send emails, make phone calls. Buy them a coffee in exchange for being allowed to pick their brain. Find out how they started, what worked for them, how they learned, and so on. Your gritty mentor could be a friend or someone you look up to, or maybe someone's uncle has a neighbor who knows somebody. A gritty mentor doesn't even need to be someone who shares your profession—they could be anyone: All they need to do is inspire you to stay gritty through their own example of *Gripping Their Grit*.

Grit Isn't Painless

Keeping yourself gritty is both a practice and a process. It's a process you've already begun. Making that long-term commitment to *Grip Your Grit* means you have to truly know yourself. It means you know how you *want* to give back to the world. It means you will cultivate an inner strength and willpower. These are all essential ingredients of grit, but your Grit Mix is still incomplete. *Gripping Your Grit* calls for a lot of on-the-job training. And some of the training, well, *sucks*. *Gripping Your Grit* is one of the few jobs where fucking up, falling down, or freaking out can actually be a sign that *you're doing it right*.

Even if you never waver in your commitment, even if you have the willpower of a god, you can still have a shitty day *while* you're *Gripping Your Grit*. You will face criticism and competition from others. You will work your ass off, lose sleep, miss meals, and sometimes still miss the mark. You'll doubt yourself. And those are all necessary and good things. Accepting criticism, at least when it's honest and constructive, is the only way you're going to get better at what you do. Competition can drive you to expect more from yourself, and it can inspire resourcefulness and creativity. Every time you doubt yourself is another opportunity to prove yourself wrong and boost your confidence.

All the people I know who have achieved anything didn't just struggle with realizing their achievements: They struggled with self-doubt. It was that little voice saying "Can I really do this?" "Am I really ready for this?" that pushed them into action. Every obstacle you have to navigate is another opportunity to *Grip Your Grit*. Duckworth describes this aspect of grittiness as staying hopeful. But what is hope, really? It's a kind of courage. And you *will* need courage, because one obstacle you will face again and again is fear.

The Thing You're Putting Off Could Be the Thing That Changes Everything

If you're putting off *Gripping Your Grit*, it's probably because you're afraid of failing or some other potential negative consequence. So what happens when you're afraid? That primitive region of your brain, the amygdala, senses your fear and sends you into Fight, Flight, or Freeze mode. *Procrastination is a form of freezing.* But you can create courage. Challenge your fear. Reality-test it. Hypothetically follow it to all of its possible outcomes. How realistic is the outcome you fear? What's the worst that could happen? What's the best that could happen? Is achieving the best worth the risk of the worst? The emotion of fear evolved in human beings to serve and protect us, and it often does. But you didn't evolve to serve fear. You evolved to *Grip Your Grit*.

The Sum of Countless Small Wins
Is an Epic Result

Gripping Your Grit isn't one huge moment of victory; *it's a collection of small wins.* Author James Altucher describes this as the 1 Percent Rule. Meaning that completing just 1 percent of something every day can set you up for colossal achievement. Over time, every small step you take and every little win you collect will lead to a quantum jump in your abilities, potential, and opportunity. On its own, an investment of 1 percent in your personal improvement doesn't seem like much. But like any good investment, that 1 percent will compound. According to Altucher, if you can improve 1 percent every week, you won't improve 365 percent in a year—you'll improve *3,800 percent*, because every day builds on the improvements of the day before.

Can you imagine committing to improving *something* in your life—a skill, a hobby, how you love, your health, for fuck's sake even your posture—by just 1 percent a day? Maybe you have an idea of what a 1 percent increase would look like tomorrow, but what do you look like a year from now at an improvement of 3,800 percent? *Gripping Your Grit* pays off in compound interest. Make your commitment, tap into your willpower, and start now.

You can even make fear work for you, because you can use it to help strengthen your commitment. Fear generates *resistance* for you to work with. Lifting weights or cycling builds up your muscles because your muscles work harder against the physical resistance provided by the weights or the bike. The resistance your fear creates is an ally. Move with it. When keeping your commitment means facing a fear, facing that fear gives you a stronger *Grip on Your Grit*.

You Are a Human Being Going Through the Process of Being Human

Now, I could start in on failure and success—how the two are connected, how to cope with failure, and how to achieve success. But there's already too much hack advice out there on success and failure. We are overfocused on them. Failure and success are not static points in time. They are repeating mile markers on your life's path—a path you cut for yourself through the process of *Gripping Your Grit*. When you stay centered in that process, it's not as easy to get lost or sidetracked by success or failure. The *process* of *Gripping Your Grit* always continues, even when that process fails to create the *product* you've been working toward.

Are you more of a Process Person or a Product Person? There's no right or wrong answer here, but it's helpful to know this about yourself. If you're a Process Person, you probably don't get as bugged by failures and setbacks as others. You perceive the Process as an ever-growing string of successes and failures, linked together. There's comfort in that, because the Process itself is indestructible. It's not that a Process Person celebrates failure or doesn't get their ego bruised. But it can be easier for them to see how a recent failure informs a future success. But the Product arrives only with success. If you're a Product Person, failure sucks extra hard because you don't just feel like you lose your center—you feel *at fault* for losing it. Who wouldn't be afraid of feeling like that? This is especially true if you're a woman.

From an early age, girls are conditioned to squelch their potential. Through socialization and enculturation, they learn to be risk averse and hyperfocused on perfection. But boys are encouraged to get dirty. We tell boys to get right back up and try again after they fall down. We give boys permission to fail while we teach girls to fear failure. Psychology professor Dr. Carol Dweck ran a study where a group of fifth-graders were given an assignment that was beyond their abilities. The results? The boys in the group charged ahead, not giving the slightest of shits if they made mistakes. But the girls held back from even trying rather than risk appearing less than perfect. In fact, the higher a girl's IQ, the more quickly she quit trying.

This carries over to the adult world. An internal report

at Hewlett-Packard found that women will usually apply for a job only if they meet 100 percent of the qualifications. Most men apply for jobs if they meet only 65 percent of the qualifications. The difference isn't gender or ability. The difference is that our culture cultivates grit in men and stifles it in women. This happens to such an extreme that it often blinds women to their own talents and potential. It's why so many women are convinced that they're not worthy and/or capable of *Gripping Their Grit*. Which is bullshit. Grit is the original equal opportunity employer.

Grip Your Grit and Your Full Potential Is Within Reach

There's a proverb that says the definition of hell is that on your last day on earth, the person you became meets the person you *could* have become. *Gripping Your Grit* is your ticket out of this hell. There is no "person you could have become": You already are that person. When I said your Process would be ongoing, I meant it in the truest sense of the word, as in never-ending. You might master one thing and then decide to change course and start doing something else, but you will always be within your Process. *You're not done until you're dead*. And that's a wonderful thing.

When my dad became a father, he made a commitment to be the kind of man who would be there to take care of his family, and there was great meaning and fulfillment in that for him (which is why he's an awesome dad). *He committed to Grip His Grit*. He fulfilled his need for meaning. Everything in his life connected to and satisfied his drive and need to care for his family. *He Gripped His Grit*. Not in some state of eternal euphoria—nobody gets that. My dad found meaning in life, something some people search for their whole lives and never find. I can't reveal the details of just how *you* will *Grip Your Grit*—that's for you to figure out. But I can tell you that you've never been more ready than you are right now. Don't be afraid. *Grip Your Grit*.

GRIP YOUR GRIT
#GOODADVICE

8

LIVE EACH DAY
LIKE IT'S YOUR LAST

Live Each Day Like It's Your Last? If I thought this was my last day alive, I wouldn't be sitting here typing. I'd do what anyone with the knowledge of their imminent death would do: I'd either be sobbing or fucking. Maybe both at the same time.

It's easy to romanticize the #BadAdvice of *Live Each Day Like It's Your Last*. Other #BadAdvice sounds like something you might hear over a cup of tea at a cozy cafe, but *Live Each Day Like It's Your Last* rides up on a motorcycle and kicks the table over. *I've got twenty-four hours and then I'm worm food, motherfuckers! YOLO! (You Only Live Once)*. It's a perfect fit with American culture's love affair with the Badass Rebel archetype. Marlon Brando. James Dean. The Fonz. (Or maybe it's a love affair with white dudes in casual jackets.)

Live Each Day Like It's Your Last is #PrivilegedAdvice targeted at comfortable First Worlders. It completely disregards your need to take care of yourself and your responsibilities to others. *Totes flaking on work today 'cuz it's *me* time #Live EachDayLikeItsMyLast #YOLO #GoFuckYourself.* Even though this #BadAdvice takes a different tone than the sappy *You Can't Love Anyone Until You Love Yourself* or the sanctimonious *Nobody Can Make You Feel Bad Without Your Permission,* its function is the same. It cons you into believing that you can outsmart pain if you don't want to feel it. *Live Each Day Like It's Your Last* tries to sell you on the sham that it's possible to go through life and never endure the pain of regret.

Ah . . . *regret.* Next to heartbreak, regret might be the emotional pain that scares us the most. And with good reason: Regret is the aftershock you feel in the present from a mistake you made in the past. And since the past is locked and unchangeable, so is the source of your regret. It's a pain that can feel unfixable. But regret is no different from any other emotion: It's a product of human evolution. It's an unavoidable feeling that you're *supposed* to experience from time to time, because it serves a survival purpose. *Regret is the emotional experience of learning from your mistakes.* You want to avoid the pain of regret, so you avoid making the same mistake that made you feel it. If you wreck your car because you were texting and driving, the regret you feel will help stop you from texting and driving in the future. (Note: Don't text and drive.) So regret isn't your enemy. It exists on your emotional spectrum for a reason.

Wasted Time Is a Universal Regret

You've probably heard some version of the saying *You only regret the things you didn't do.* Google it and you'll find multiple versions falsely attributed to famous authors, movies, and poets. What matters more than who said it is *why* this saying is so popular: It affirms a common fear. No one wants to spend their last moments wondering how life might have been better if they hadn't done this or chosen to do that. Nobody wants their final realization in life to be *I blew it.* Still, it's impossible to know how and when a particular choice you make in the present plants a seed of regret in your future. Which is where *Live Each Day Like It's Your Last* comes in, offering you the Capital-A Answer for how to avoid regret in life: *DO EVERYTHING! NOW! ALL THE TIME! LIVE EACH DAY LIKE IT'S YOUR LAST, MOFO!* What a load of shit. So where the hell did this come from, anyway?

You Can't Live Each Day Like It's Your Last, but You Can Live So That on Your Last Day, You Feel Good About What You've Done

One version of this #BadAdvice, "Live each day like it's your last, 'cause one day you gonna be right," is attributed to two legit American rebels: Muhammad Ali and Ray Charles.

Some people credit the controversial Australian folk hero Breaker Morant with the saying. But this #BadAdvice was around long before them. The Roman emperor Marcus Aurelius wrote, "To live each day as though one's last, never flustered, never apathetic, never attitudinizing—here is perfection of character." Not as punchy as our modern version, but criticizing the emperor back then could mean living your last day running from lions in the Colosseum. A little less than a hundred years before Marcus Aurelius, the Roman poet Horace coined the famous aphorism *Carpe diem*: "Seize the day."

But neither the emperor nor the poet is guilty of creating #BadAdvice. Aurelius's "perfection of character" is found in serenity: "Never flustered, never apathetic, never attitudinizing." In other words, on your last day alive, you're not losing your shit, you still give a shit, and you're not giving anybody shit. "Performing every act of your life as if it were your last" means being focused and deliberate, because you want to be sure that the last thing you do has meaning. *Carpe diem* has been even more misunderstood. In fact, it is only part of the last line of an ode that reads, "Seize the day, put very little trust in tomorrow." Horace is saying that since you don't know what will happen tomorrow, do all you can to get ready for it today. Which is the exact fucking *opposite* of what *Live Each Day Like It's Your Last* tells you to do. SPQR, bitchez. (SPQR is the Latin abbreviation for "Senate and People of Rome," according to my history nerd co-writer, Paul Feldman.)

Each Day Holds No More or Less Meaning than You Give It

Live Each Day Like It's Your Last is #BadAdvice because it wants you to believe that you'll find the path to lifelong fulfillment through instant gratification, without ever having to risk regret. *Enjoy everything to the fullest, right fucking now!* But living life to the fullest comes with creating purpose, meaning, and fulfillment when you connect with other people. That's a lifelong process, not an instantaneous one. So this #BadAdvice can create a pathologically isolating mindset. It's hard to stay centered in your connection to and impact on others if your prime directive is *Gotta get mine today because I'm gone tomorrow. #YOLO!* The impact on modern society is painfully obvious: The fossil fuel, tobacco, and firearms industries are all living each day like it's their last, with no thought of future generations.

#YOLO is a mindset that makes it easier to be an asshole, because it keeps you focused *only* on yourself in the present. You never consider anyone else at any other time. It means the same thing at the personal level as it does at the corporate: *Fuck you and fuck me.* Which is why following this #BadAdvice means saying *Fuck you* to your future—because you don't plan on showing up for it. Still, though, that fear of *blowing it*, that fear of dying with a basketful of regrets next to your bed, is very real. So let's stare that fear down together, right now. I happen to have on hand one of the most effective remedies for fear: *information*. If you're afraid of potential deathbed regrets and want to avoid them, *Why not find out what dying people actually regret?*

Your Days Are Limited, But Filled with Infinite Richness

Regret can turn us into ghosts long before we're dead. Bronnie Ware was a hospice nurse before writing her book *The Top Five Regrets of the Dying: A Life Transformed by the Dearly Departing* (2013). Ware observed that her patients most often regretted living their lives to satisfy others at the expense of finding their own fulfillment and satisfaction. They regretted working too much. They regretted never learning to express their feelings. (And by extension, they never learned to satisfy their needs.) They regretted losing connection with old friends. Another common regret Ware described was, "I wish that I had let myself be happier."

Now wait a hot second. Haven't I spent this entire book railing against the idea that you can choose to let yourself feel things? Haven't I spent this entire book hammering home how crucial it is to be aware of your connection with and responsibility to the people in your life? Is this the big reveal of Dr. V's *Bad Advice*, where you discover that I, Dr. V, am in fact full of shit? (Spoiler alert! I'm not—at least not in this regard.)

The thing is, Ware uses the statement "I wish I would have let myself be happier" to explain her patients' regret that their fear of change and/or being too attached to familiar dysfunction had held them back in life. But would *Live Each Day Like It's Your Last* help you avoid those regrets? Well . . . maybe. If you thought you were going to die tomorrow, you probably wouldn't be worried about meeting anyone's expectations. You'd skip work to go fuck off with your friends and Live Each Day like you had a corporate endorsement from an Energy Drink. Forget that it's impossible to *Live Each Day Like It's Your Last*, and let's just pretend you could. It'd be like celebrating your birthday every day. Eventually it would become routine and lose meaning, bringing you back to where you started. That's not a sustainable way to live: Ask any recovering drug addict.

You know, I almost left this chapter out just because *Live Each Day Like It's Your Last* in fact *does* have a slight potential to be helpful. Recently, I've had a sharpened awareness of the fact that my time *is* limited. Maybe it's because I've gotten a little older, maybe it's because I've lost people close to me; but somehow, any given day being my last doesn't seem like such a stretch. So before bed I've begun asking myself, *Did I get the most I could out of today? What would I want to do differently? How do I want to feel tomorrow?* At first, I thought I was asking myself whether I had lived that day as if it were my last. But then I realized NO. The questions I was really asking myself were, *Did I live today to the fullest? Will what I did today give me something to build on tomorrow?* Instead of being focused on doing as much as I could before I croaked, I was preparing for the future. Instead of living each day like it was my last, I'm living each day as if it's just the beginning. It's a philosophy reflected in this chapter's #GoodAdvice.

Live Each Day Like
It's Your Own #GOODADVICE

Before I go any further, can I just share something with you? *I fucking hate self-help books.* They tell you how to live your life. They tell you what to do and how to do it. So any time I offer you #GoodAdvice or any other suggestion, know that *that is all they are:* suggestions. You own your life. The decisions are yours. I have no answers for you—you need to find them for yourself. At best, I offer potential paths to help you find those answers.

It matters that you find your own answers and create your meaning in life because doing so will give you a sense of agency, empowerment, and ownership over *your* time, *your* days, and *your* life. That is what it means to *Live Each Day Like It's Your Own.* Your days are yours, as long as you remember they are. This doesn't mean that some days you won't have to do shit you'd rather not do, or that you'll never have to endure anything unpleasant, or that you'll always understand the why and how of everything that happens in life. What it does mean is that you are not living your life on autopilot. You aren't "going through the motions." Your life isn't reduced to a robotic repetition of habitual behaviors.

This is deliberate living, where life is an experience that you create "on purpose." When you *Live Each Day Like It's Your Own*, you don't expect immunity from regret. You are still a human being who will occasionally fuck up and regret it when you do. But what you *won't* do is reach the end of your life and face the heartbreaking realization that you wasted your precious, all-too-finite time here. *Living Each Day Like It's Your Own* means that you recognize the purpose and meaning behind all that you do. You understand that each day of your life is another stone laid on your life's path. Some are smoother than others, but they are all supporting you in your journey forward.

But forward to where? It wasn't so long ago I couldn't answer that question (and there are times I *still* can't). So you and I both better fucking figure out where this all is going before it's over. (After all, this is the last chapter of the book.)

The Only Thing You Want to Do on Your Deathbed Is Die; Take Care of Everything Else Before You Get There

In 2009, artist Candy Chang lost someone she loved very much. The death of a loved one is always devastating, and Chang struggled with sadness and depression while she grieved. But in her grief, she found gratitude for her own life and the time she still had left to live. She also gained new clarity about and perspective on what was important in life and wanted to share this with others. So Chang, along with some help from her friends, converted the exterior wall of an abandoned house near her home in New Orleans into a giant chalkboard. In the top left corner in large letters is the statement *Before I die* . . . Beneath it are rows and rows of the same, fill-in-the-blank sentence: *Before I die, I want to* ____. Overnight, passersby filled the entire wall with responses ranging from funny to profound to heartrending.

Before I die, I want to hold her one more time.

Before I die, I want to love and be loved.

Before I die, I want to be tried for piracy.

Before I Die became a global phenomenon—since 2009, people throughout the Americas, Europe, Asia, and the Pacific have filled in the blanks on their own *Before I Die* walls. In an interview with San Francisco's SOMArts, Chang said:

> *Death is something we're often discouraged to talk about or even think about. . . . Beyond the tragic truth of mortality lies a bright calm that reminds me of my place in the world. When I think about death, the mundane things that stress me out are reduced to their small and rightful place. The things that matter most to me become big and crisp again. Regularly*

contemplating death . . . is a powerful tool to restore perspective and remember the things that make your life personally meaningful.

So set this book aside for a moment and fill in the blank: *Before I die I want to ____.*

Don't Get So Busy
You Never Get Anything Done

Okay. You've contemplated death. Now that you've reflected on that terrifying idea of Not Being Here (because you're dead), shift gears and focus on your present situation: *You Are Alive. You Are Here.* So practice being present. Don't take that too lightly: Being present is a pretty tall order when you're always under pressure to be *busy*.

We live in a workaholic culture; Americans work longer hours, take less time off, and retire later than just about anyone else in the industrialized world. To be *busy* is something to strive for—as if you've achieved some kind of spiritual enlightenment that the un-busy losers of the world will never know. "You may not speak to Carol. She is busy." People declare they're *busy* like it's some kind of badge of honor.

But it's not really about being *busy*; it's about what we've made the word "busy" mean. *Busy* means *unavailable*. So, if you constantly project and perceive yourself as busy, where does that leave you emotionally? How can you connect with anyone or yourself? *How can you be present if you're perpetually unavailable?* So how can you cultivate an appreciation of being un-busy? Make a commitment to *respect your quiet moments.*

Find Some Quiet and You'll Hear Everything

What does it mean to respect your quiet moments? Don't strive to fill them needlessly. If there's nothing to do, it's okay to do nothing. There's a difference between working to get ahead, and working only to *feel* like you're getting ahead. The only way to know the difference is to be in an un-busy state. You don't need to be meditating on a mountaintop; just slow down. If your responsibilities and expectations start to feel overwhelming, create a quiet moment for yourself. Find the time and space to be alone. Just do nothing, and give the machinery in your head a rest. As much as possible, don't let this process be interrupted (exceptions being emergencies, of course). This is *your* time; you're entitled to use it for yourself.

Creating and respecting your quiet moments gives you a break from the inevitable hectic, dare I say, *busy* times of life. You could even carve out a regularly scheduled time in your day to be un-busy. Whether that's closing your eyes and breathing deeply or just disconnecting from any and all screens, make it a regular practice to create and respect your quiet moments. In other words, *make a commitment to being un-busy*. And if somebody tries to muscle in on your quiet moments . . . just tell them you're busy. You're allowed to; you're *Living Each Day Like It's Your Own*.

Clutter Where You Live Will Clutter How You Think

But what if you're *not* busy? Don't worry. I've got some shit for you to do. When I was in high school, I worked at a fast-food joint. My manager's favorite thing to say was, "If you got time to lean, you got time to clean." I still hear that shit ringing in my ears today, and it applies here. Part of *Living Each Day Like It's Your Own* is making yourself feel like the physical space you live in is your own. Do you live surrounded by clutter? Do you have drawers or closets you just don't go into? *Reclaim your physical space*. Clean out your closet, garage, and any other place you keep shit, and give what you can to people in need.

On a metaphysical level, I'm a firm believer that when you clear away clutter and make room in your physical space, you also open up room in your psychological space. Make that your deliberate intention, and you will transform the chore of tidying up into an action with much deeper meaning. Besides, there's scientific proof that doing this shit's good for you. Researchers have found that people who consistently keep their living spaces tidy exhibit better emotional and physical health. So get rid of everything that doesn't serve you. Pass on what you no longer need to someone who needs it. Reclaim your space so you can start *Living Each Day Like It's Your Own.*

Even If You Haven't Found an Outlet, You *Are* Creative

If I told you to *Be Creative*, you'd probably think I was asking you to write a poem, draw a picture, or do some other activity one could classify as artsy-fartsy. It's true that artsy-fartsy things are creative, but they're not the only avenues of creative expression available to you. (Of course, if you hear the call of the artsy-fartsy, heed it.) Creativity is your innate human ability to express yourself through the change you create in the world around you. You are absolutely capable of creating real and immediate change in your life. It can be as simple as changing what you wear, what you have for dinner tonight, or the route you take to work tomorrow. One change leads to another, and you may find that the smallest action creates a domino effect you never could have foreseen. *Express your creativity.* In this way you are creating difference in what could otherwise feel like a never-ending sea of sameness in your life. But more important, you're tapping into the fearless part of your heart that never dies. *That* is the gift of *Living Each Day Like It's Your Own.*

Be Deliberate:
There Is No Undo Button in Life

If you're going to *Live Each Day Like It's Your Own*, you have to be able to tell the difference between the pain of paying your dues and the pain of selling yourself out. Let's be honest here. From time to time, we all have to do or go through shit we don't want to. Trying to evade that certainty is a first step on the road to #BadAdvice. Those unpleasant experiences often help you because you grit your teeth, get through it, and chalk it up to *paying your dues*. Struggle isn't always a bad thing, it's often the price of forward motion.

But there's a difference between having to do something you don't want to do, and doing something you hate. How can you tell the difference? *You'll know you're doing something you hate when you hate yourself for doing it.* What this all boils down to is being sure not to ignore your conscience. When you *Live Each Day Like It's Your Own*, you don't expect to enjoy everything you do, *but it does require that you do everything on purpose.*

So just what the hell do I mean when I say you should *do everything on purpose?* I mean that you need to recognize the importance and impact of everything you do, every day of your life. If you *Live Each Day Like It's Your Own*, then you will be deliberate and purposeful in how you spend those days. Recognize that each day you live is *yours*, and it's something you have in limited quantity. Your days are the building blocks of *Your Life,* and your life will only hold the meaning you decide to infuse it with. So every day of your life, *do something important.* It doesn't matter what that thing is, as long as *you* believe and feel it's important. Do something that feels meaningful, something that gives you a sense of purpose in the world.

Maybe you'll do that thing at work, maybe you'll do it on the way to work, maybe you'll do it waiting in line somewhere. Stay aware of and receptive to the opportunities that present themselves to you each day—opportunities to connect with someone and help them get what they need. Something as small as holding the door open for a stranger might be all it takes. Do something important and meaningful every day, and you'll discover a reward of *Living Each Day Like It's Your Own* that pays out over time. Instead of wondering at the end of your life *What did it all mean?,* you'll know you've lived a life rich in meaning. *You'll know that you mattered.* Your time is limited, *but you still have time.* Your time is yours. Your life is yours. *You* choose the meaning it will have, not just on one day, but every day. Because when you *Live Each Day Like It's Your Own,* you move closer to immortality.

If You Want to Live Forever, Inspire Someone

In his Pulitzer Prize–winning book *The Denial of Death* (1973), cultural anthropologist Ernest Becker suggested that humans evolved a behavior to cope with their fear of death. He said that humans pursue "immortality projects"—or "something that we feel will outlast our time on earth." For some people, their immortality project takes the form of religion or spirituality. Some people pour themselves into a career as a way to feel plugged into something bigger than themselves. But an immortality project doesn't have to be positive to be functional. Becker also believed that racism, genocide, and war were the result of conflicting immortality projects. If different groups of people believe theirs is the One True Faith, then anyone refusing to accept that One True Faith is a threat to the immortality projects of others (and by extension, their whole defense mechanism against death). This could help explain today's caustic political climate. *It's not really your politics that bug me, it's just that your opinion invalidates my existence. So I'll now channel my existential panic into an epic online rage-sesh of trolling. YOLO!*

So how do you create a positive and effective immortality project for yourself?

You Matter—More Than You Know

A never-ending stream of selfies. Someone's initials scrawled with a Sharpie on a bus seat. The Great Pyramid of Giza in Egypt. They all carry the same message of *I was here* and the same subtext of *I matter*. This is the message of all immortality projects. For *your* immortality project to be effective, *you* need to be the primary intended receiver of that message, not the rest of the world.

So how do you, a twenty-first-century human, create a sustainable and effective immortality project? Start with the inarguable and scientifically verified fact that *you matter*. You matter because on this planet that you share with billions of other humans, *you* are the only you. The specific combination of genetics, environment, and experience that makes you who you are has never happened before, and it will never happen again. And you almost didn't happen. Dr. Ali Binazir, author of *The Tao of Dating* (2010), expanded on an idea popularized by self-help author Mel Robbins. Taking into account all the different variables of life, Binazir crunched the numbers and concluded that there was only a one in 400 trillion chance of you even *existing*. There are things that only you will say, ideas that only you will have, and people who only you will move in a unique way.

And that's no small number of people, by the way. According to one algorithm, you probably know around 600 people. And those 600 people know 600 people, so now that's 36,000 lives you could potentially make a difference in. And according to infographic author Anna Vital, you will probably meet, if only in passing, around 80,000 people. You are a being who beat insurmountable odds even to exist, with the potential to affect a total of 440,000 people. *You matter.* You matter because so much depends on your existence to exist. You are irreplaceable. And because you matter so much, it's vital for you to create a connection with something bigger than yourself. The reason is because we, the Rest of the Whole Fucking World, *need* you present and functioning at optimal levels. We need you to maximize your direct influence on all those hundreds of thousands of people. *The world needs you to Live Each Day Like It's Your Own.*

Regret Is a Moment; You Are Ongoing

German philosopher Friedrich Nietzsche wrote "He who has a why to live can bear almost any how." The immortality project you create for yourself works on regret the way vitamin C works on a cold: Your immortality project can't cure regret, but it can help you process and move through it. This is because a positive and effective immortality project helps fuel a very specific mechanism of your mind: *Your psychological immune system.* Researchers Daniel Gilbert and Jane Ebert describe your psychological immune system as your psyche's built-in ability to find ways to justify, rationalize, and otherwise make peace with a situation you no longer have control over. You're able to perceive yourself in a larger context. Without denying the regret you feel, you're still aware that who and what you are is too vast to be defined by any single moment, action, or decision. Your psychological immune system is the immediate, in-the-moment payoff of your immortality project. It's what ultimately helps you to remember that *you are not your regrets.*

Regret Is a Lesson Mistaken for Punishment

Scientific data suggest that you feel regret most strongly when you think you can do something about a situation. And the feeling of regret is even stronger when you *know* what needs to be done. This is called the "the Opportunity Principle." One possible explanation for the Opportunity Principle could be that the stronger an emotion is, the more likely it is to motivate you to do something. But even when you can't do anything about what you regret, it can still be of benefit.

Have you ever found yourself thinking, "If I only did/didn't do whatever, I wouldn't be feeling this shitty regret now"? Psychologists call this "counterfactual thinking," and it's how regret works as an emotional reinforcement to keep you from making the same mistake again. The #BadAdvice of *Live Each Day Like It's Your Last* won't let you engage your regret or learn from it because it cons you into believing that regret is punishment for wasting your life. So this #BadAdvice cuts you off from information that will help you *Live Each Day Like It's Your Own* because it stops you from experiencing your life in its totality. But *Live Each Day Like It's Your Last* denies more than your regrets; *it denies what you have to be grateful for.*

Gratitude: Seeking Out the Good Already Present in Your Life

The #BadAdvice of *Live Each Day Like It's Your Last* can never fulfill its promise to help you avoid regret and get the most out of life. Minimizing regret and finding fulfillment only come when you're able to find real meaning in life, and there is no shortcut to meaning. The path you need to take is slower and more contemplative: the path of gratitude.

Gratitude is the opposite of "taking things for granted." It is a simple but profound shift in perception. Don't confuse the practice of gratitude with trying to "look on the bright side" of a shitty situation. Sometimes a shitty situation *is* a shitty situation. Practicing gratitude acknowledges the reality of your problem, but it also widens your focus. You're able to take in the decidedly nonshitty elements of your life. Gratitude is a reminder that this is a life of multiple, not singular, truths. *You can have a bad day and a fantastic life at the same time.*

The art of practicing gratitude reveals the priceless treasures hidden in the everyday of your life. These are the things you can't live without, but their constant presence tricks you into perceiving them as mundane. Instead of fixating on what is absent, you move your focus to what *is* present: the verifiable, concrete good in your life. You remind yourself that your life, even *all* life, is the result of an infinite number of one-in-a-million miracles happening daily. Your breath is something to be grateful for. Your heartbeat is something to be grateful for. Every thought in your brain is something to be grateful for. The undeniable reality that your days are yours, and the meaning of those days is yours to create, is something to be grateful for. *Living Each Day Like It's Your Own* is something to be grateful for. *Live Each Day Like It's Your Own, Because It Is.*

The practice and experience of gratitude create an awareness that you exist in an unconditionally supportive universe. On his show *Cosmos*, astrophysicist and All-Around Badass Neil deGrasse Tyson said, "We are all connected to each other biologically, to the earth chemically, and to the rest of the universe atomically. . . . We are in the universe and the universe is in us." So even if you have doubts about your personal immortality project, know that you are effortlessly connected, *at a fucking atomic level*, with the universe, the original Immortality Project. You are made of stuff forged in the heart of stars. You're stronger than you think.

You May Never Know How Much There Is to Be Thankful For, and *That's* Something to Be Thankful For

Gratitude isn't "settling" or allowing yourself to become complacent, either. Gratitude is both a practice and an emotion. Beyond shifting your perception from negative to positive, practicing gratitude is an act of self-empowerment. You are taking deliberate action to look for and acknowledge the good that exists in your life. When you acknowledge the good, you'll realize that the universe is working for you (and not the narcissistic "Universe" that "manifests" to twenty-something white kids at Malibu Yoga Retreats. I mean the *real* universe. The thing that unconditionally provides you with oxygen, gravity, Wi-Fi, and other shit you might take for granted but would definitely notice the second it went missing). Recognizing where you are supported and strong gives you a source to draw strength from. You are perfectly positioned and equipped to move ahead into whatever greatness is coming next, or to reach out and claim whatever is waiting for you.

This may not always be easy, but that's okay because something not being easy is not a deal breaker for you—not when you remember that you are exactly where you need to be and you have everything you need *in this moment*. The practice of gratitude not only highlights the existing good in your life, it's been shown to create good things in measurable amounts.

Gratitude Is One of the Few Things You Can Be Filled with That Makes Room for More

Now, I realize that a conversation about gratitude can easily devolve into some cotton-candy self-help bullshit: sweet, fluffy words that have jack-shit to do with the reality of your life. So I'll balance out candy sweetness with some hardcore vegetables: Time for one last helping of science, bitchezzzzz! Dr. Robert Emmons has made the psychology of gratitude the focus of his work. In a study conducted with Dr. Mike McCullough, Emmons found that people who made a regular practice of gratitude showed a 25 percent greater level of happiness than those who regularly listed the negative things in their lives. The gratitude-focused group also felt physically healthier and generally exercised more. These results were echoed in a 2013 study that revealed a state of good general physical health in people who regularly practiced gratitude. Why is this? When you appreciate something, you take good care of it. So when you appreciate yourself, you take good care of yourself—exercising regularly, seeing a doctor regularly, etc.

The practice of gratitude also affects the brain. In 2015, Prathik Kini and colleagues recruited people suffering from anxiety and/or depression. For three weeks, their subjects were guided in a practice of regular gratitude (writing thank-you letters). Two weeks later, the same people reported feeling increased levels of gratitude and improved mental health. If you're still not impressed, Kini's subjects continued to experience the benefits of their three-week gratitude practice *three months after the study ended*. That's a damn good return on an investment. Gratitude is a tremendous generator for the infinite potential good you carry inside you, and it takes just a nudge to activate it. In fact, sometimes all you need to do is *remember to try*.

Dr. Sonja Lyubomirsky has conducted extensive research on gratitude and its relationship to people's happiness and enjoyment of life. In one study, she and a colleague found that people who would be considered "happy," people living fulfilling and joyful lives, were *deliberate* about creating that fulfillment and joy. They achieved that through a commitment to daily reflection on what they had to be grateful for. The gratitude they felt didn't necessarily come from something immediately obvious, like material wealth. Much of these people's gratitude appeared to originate from simply *remembering* to look for things to be grateful for as much as it did from actually having those things to appreciate.

Gratitude allows you to rediscover a sense of awe for the everyday wonders around you. Gratitude is what clears your way toward *Living Each Day Like It's Your Own*. And you can start in a comfortable place. Start while you're in bed.

Opening Your Eyes in the Morning Qualifies for the First "Thank You" of the Day

There's a certain moment after you wake in the morning, but before you open your eyes. You're conscious, but your day has yet to begin. For almost my entire life, I skipped through this moment without thinking about it. I woke up, opened my eyes, and began my usual search for three things: *robe, glasses, whatever I'm trying to do instead of smoke a cigarette first thing in the morning*. And I'll tell you what, committing to a daily practice of gratitude is how I quit smoking. Every morning, I always remembered to be grateful for my health. That's when I realized, *If I'm so grateful for my health, why the fuck am I still smoking?* In that moment I realized my gratitude for my health outweighed my desire to smoke. Quitting wasn't easy—God knows I had failed at it soooooooo many times already. The difference this time was gratitude. The feeling and practice of gratitude gave me support and strength when I needed it. I still maintain my commitment to my morning practice of gratitude. It saved my life. With my eyes still closed, I focus on identifying five things to be grateful for. And without our ever meeting, I'm *positive* you can do the same.

How Much Do You Take for Granted Things That Others Would Call Luxuries?

Take an inventory right now of things to feel grateful for that someone else might consider an unattainable luxury or even a superpower. I'll help you get started: *You can read.* Because of this skill, you're empowered to seek out your own answers without relying on others to relay information to you. Maybe being able to read doesn't sound like that big of a deal, but it is. According to a 2013 survey, *thirty-two million Americans* can't read. Thirty-two million people are cut off and excluded from an aspect of life that it's hard for you and me to imagine surviving without. Boom. That's one thing to be grateful for. Go ahead and add the people you love and trust to the list. That's three things. You can be grateful for having the time to read this book, for the place you live, for waking up, the breakfast you ate, your breath, your heartbeat, and for having the presence of mind to even *remember* to practice gratitude. There, I gave you a two-day head start with ten things you can be grateful for. Now you try. Identify five more things to be grateful for.

As your gratitude reveals itself to you, don't forget to recognize the active role you play in making it manifest in your life. If you're grateful for a relationship, recognize the contributions you make to that relationship to sustain it. If you're grateful for the work you do, the home you have, your health, and so on, recognize the responsibilities you fulfill to maintain all those things. Even if it's something as simple as appreciating the beauty of the day, recognize the awareness and presence of mind you have that allow you to perceive that simple beauty.

In this way, you begin to understand the direct impact you have in helping good things materialize in your life. Put this deliberate practice of gratitude in action before you even open your eyes, and you will begin each day in a place of positive, life-affirming empowerment. It's a power with a firm foundation in reality. It's something reliable to fall back on. You will start each day with a renewed connection with what is best in yourself. Not only that, *You Will Live Each Day Like It's Your Own.*

You Live More Than Once:
Your Actions Echo Forever

You can even buy gratitude—for the price of a stamp. When was the last time you got a letter in the mail? An actual letter, handwritten by a human being whom you know and care about? If you can't remember the 1990s, maybe you've never even had that experience. If you have, you know how great a letter can make you feel. It's a physical manifestation of someone's thoughts for you. You meant enough to someone that it was worth their time to write the letter and send it. It's tangible proof that you matter to someone. Getting a sincere, handwritten thank-you note can carry even more meaning, as it says that not only you, but what you did or what you gave, matter. So I suggest this: Once a week, send an actual physical thank-you note to someone. It could be to the friend who was there when you needed them last week, or to the Seventh-Grade Teacher Who Changed Everything for You.

Sending a thank-you note also creates an opportunity for the person receiving it to experience gratitude. In a study published in 2015, researchers Lisa Williams and Monica Bartlett found that someone receiving a thank-you note from a new acquaintance made them more likely to reach out to the sender, in the hopes of further deepening their new connection and friendship. When that happens, *you* have helped someone else feel good and potentially access all the benefits of gratitude. You've made an impact on the world for the better. You've connected to something bigger than yourself. You've added another facet to your immortality project: When you inspire feelings in others, they are inspired to act. Their actions inspire feelings in *other* people and so on—your influence spirals out across the planet forever. In this way, when you *Live Each Day Like It's Your Own*, you live forever.

A well-lived life unfolds one day at a time. Regret in and of itself is not a bad thing. It exists on your emotional spectrum for a reason, and like anything else on a spectrum, it comes in more than one color. The #BadAdvice of *Live Each Day Like It's Your Last* tries to pass itself off as a shield against regret, but what it really shields you from is your own potential for finding meaning and fulfillment in life. As an emotion, regret is both inevitable and meaningful: It's nature's insurance policy that you will learn from your mistakes. *Living Each Day Like It's Your Own* won't save you from regret, but that's okay, because nothing can. But this #GoodAdvice can yield near-limitless opportunities for you to find connection, fulfillment, and meaning. Each day adds another invaluable layer to your immortality project. The sum total of *Living Each Day Like It's Your Own* is *Living Your* Life *Like It's Your Own*, and it is. *Do it*. Make your time on this planet the lifelong experience of the singular, undeniable, and ever-expanding potential that is *You*.

LIVE EACH DAY LIKE IT'S YOUR OWN

#GOODADVICE

(There. I fixed you. Thank you for reading this book.)

SO WHAT NOW?

Well, all right! You finished this book. Hugs and high-fives all around! And now that you've finished reading it, you might be wondering the same thing I was when I finished writing it: *So what now?*

What now? You get back out there and really *live*. Don't put it off, because *the world needs you to live*. Granted, the world is the same fucked-up, imperfect place it was when you first picked up this book. But you aren't. Even if you don't think you've changed at all, *you have*. And just how the fuck would I know that? After all, unless some crazy, unforeseen shit went down between the first page and now, you and I still haven't even met. I don't know your name, what you look like, or how to find you on Twitter. So how can I be so certain you've changed? Because there's one more thing I *do* know about you: You just finished reading a self-help book called

Bad Advice. That tells me you now know and understand more about the how, what, and why of your emotions and your needs and who you really are. Because your perception and awareness of yourself have changed, *you have changed too*. When you began reading this book, you began changing yourself.

You've changed because you now know that you are never "wrong" or "fucked-up" for feeling anything. You've changed because you know your emotions are messengers of survival, not signs of weakness. You understand that while nobody *wants* to feel hurt, betrayed, heartbroken, disappointed, or any other shade of shitty, sometimes *you need to feel those things*. Pain, whether it's physical or emotional, is a signal that your status quo needs to change. That can mean pulling your hand out of the fire that's burning it, or pulling yourself out of (or changing) a situation that's burning you. You're different now because you've replaced fear with understanding—the understanding that *every* possible combination and variation of hues on your emotional spectrum exist to help you survive and thrive.

You've changed because you know that *everything* you feel is another thread of connection that runs between you, other people, and the world you share. How you feel is equally rooted in the tangible chemistry of your body and the intangibility of what you feel in your heart. You now see your emotions for what they are: a transcendent experience. Only #BadAdvice would tell you that a transcendent experience is something you want to avoid. And only a fucked-up

society would tell you you're fucked-up for simply *feeling*.
You've changed because you know that even at their most
painful, your emotions aren't monsters you need to hide
from or dirty secrets for you to carry in shame and silence.
And if this book changes nothing else for you, what I want
most is for you to come away certain of this one truth: *There
is nothing wrong with you.*

I'm not a religious person. Calling me a practicing agnos-
tic would be a stretch. Still, more than I know or believe it, I
just *feel* that there is something more to the lives we live than
what we can immediately sense or perceive. Call that God,
the Tao, the Force, Love, the Laws of Physics, or whatever
you want. Embedded in that feeling of knowing is the certainty that you, for lack of a better phrase, are a Child of God.
Countless years of evolution and chance events conspired to
create *you*, and you were created in perfection. Right now in
this moment, you are perfect. A year ago, you were perfect. A
year from now, you will still be perfect. That ongoing perfection is possible only because Tomorrow's Perfect doesn't have
to match Today's Perfect. And sometimes making the shift
from past to present perfect can't happen without sweat and
tears. (Let's be optimistic and leave out the blood.) That was
true before you read this book, and it will remain true long
after you finish it. Like I said before: The world is the same;
what's changed is *you*. You're not just going to live, but you're
going change how you live in the world.

You're now armed with #GoodAdvice instead of being lost
in #BadAdvice. You don't seek out pain, conflict, or problems,

but you don't run from them either. You've learned to choose courage over cowering. That courage is based in true self-confidence, self-trust, self-awareness, and self-knowledge. You understand that no matter how strong any emotion may be, it will never be bigger than you. You can trust yourself to experience all that you feel, without the fear of *becoming* what you feel.

My parting #GoodAdvice to you is to *Trust yourself to live.* Trust yourself to live in a way that honors who you are, what you need, and how you feel. Your example could one day provide someone with the inspiration they didn't know they were waiting for. Trust yourself to live.

Trust yourself to live courageously and deliberately. You can if you want to. You can because beyond recognizing your emotions as messengers of survival, you also know that they are always temporary: They roll like clouds across the sky of your psyche. But centered in that sky is the constant-shining star that is *you.* Like any other star in the sky, you are always perfect. You are always changing. And you will always shine with a light uniquely your own.

Always.

ACKNOWLEDGMENTS

To my below conspirators in *Bad Advice*, I offer my boundless gratitude, and/or a gift card to the closest discount adult beverage store of your choice. Let the "Thank Yous" begin:

Thank you to my editor, Libby Edelson: Thank you for believing in me and this book, even when my own belief in one or both of those things wavered. Your insight, critique, and perspective were invaluable throughout this process. Your authentic, unshakeable passion for this book is unforgettable. You don't know this; but when I can think of nothing good about myself, I reread the very first email you sent to my agent regarding *Bad Advice*. In fact, I printed it out, and now show it to people I'm arguing with as concrete proof that *someone* likes me and my work. (Mostly, I show it to myself.)

To my agent, Nicole Tourtelot: Thank you for helping me fulfill my lifetime goal of writing a book and having someone pay me to do it. You are not just a literary agent, you're an agent of change, an agent of purpose, and an agent of action.

Thank you for showing up at my house, lighting a fire under my ass to write the proposal for *Bad Advice*, and for keeping that fire blazing for the next one. (There's gonna be a Next One, right?)

To my co-writer, Paul Feldman: For the past ten years, you've helped me hone a literary voice that I am deeply proud of and that others depend on. You help translate my multidimensional ideas, words, expressions, and feelings into the singular dimension of words. More than just that, you are my friend. One of my dearest friends, as we are both in each other's typo confidence. (Learn to spell "experience," ya schmuck.)

To my parents and siblings: Thank you for damaging me just enough to make me funny, yet being supportive enough to keep me motivated. You guys are the best.

To my husband, Matthew: Of everyone on this list, I have the most to say to you, yet the fewest words to do it . . . because words fall short of expressing all that I feel for you. Words are finite and limiting. The love I feel for you is boundless, immeasurable, and unending. But I'm still gonna try. Love is as close as humans get to creating something perfect. I've never gotten closer to that perfection with anyone but you. I thank you for your limitless tolerance, unending patience, and quiet strength. I thank you for showing me how to love and be loved. I thank you for going along with every crazy idea I've ever had, which usually entailed you giving up something or giving something. I thank you for teaching our children courage, strength, and empathy.

I thank you for cherishing me every single day: love notes found in my pockets; phone calls from airplanes far away; sexy glances, touches, and kisses to let me know that after twenty-one years, I still rock your world. (And you still rock mine, btw.) You never set out to change me but you did; I am forever changed by your adoring love and my life would be empty and meaningless without you. And when I can think of nothing good about myself, I take solace in knowing that you, this incredible brilliant star, loves me unconditionally. I love you. I love you. I love you.

To my sons, Ledger and Laith, Baby Anjelica, and to every kid everywhere: You carry within you stuff forged in the heart of stars. May your ever-burning light never be dimmed by anyone's #BadAdvice.

NOTES

1. Just Be Yourself

9: *eight million people struggle with eating disorders:* "Eating
Disorder Statistics," ANAD, National Association of Anorexia
Nervosa and Associated Disorders, www.anad.org/education
-and-awareness/about-eating-disorders/eating-disorders
-statistics/, accessed June 29, 2018.

9: *LGBTQIA kids remain at greater risk of suicide:* Katherine
Schreiber, "Why Are Suicide Rates Higher Among LGBTQ
Youth?," *Psychology Today*, October 12, 2017, https://www
.psychologytoday.com/us/blog/the-truth-about-exercise-addiction
/201710/why-are-suicide-rates-higher-among-lgbtq-youth.

12: *"They don't know what they're doing":* Erich C. Dierdorff and
Robert S. Rubin, "Research: We're Not Very Self-Aware, Especially at Work," *Harvard Business Review*, March 12, 2015,
https://www.hbr.org/2015/03/research-were-not-very-self-aware
-especially-at-work.

13: *the stories . . . are not true:* "Etymology of the 'F-Word,'" Snopes
.com, updated February 21, 2016, https://www.snopes.com/fact
-check/what-the-fuck/.

20: *it's actually good for your health, too:* Tori Rodriguez, "Writing
Can Help Injuries Heal Faster," *Scientific American*, November 1,
2013, https://www.scientificamerican.com/article/writing-can
-help-injuries-heal-faster/; Alanna Ketler, "Scientific Studies

Show How Writing in a Journal Can Actually Benefit Your
Emotional & Physical Well-Being," Collective Evolution, January
23, 2017, https://www.collective-evolution.com/2017/01/23
/scientific-studies-show-how-writing-in-a-journal-can-actually
-benefit-your-emotional-physical-well-being/; Michael Grothaus,
"Why Journaling Is Good for Your Health (and 8 Tips to Get
Better)," Fast Company, January 29, 2015, https://www.fast
company.com/3041487/8-tips-to-more-effective-journaling-for
-health.

23: *an increase in feelings of confidence and self-acceptance:* "UCI
Study Links Selfies, Happiness," UCI News, September 13, 2016,
news.uci.edu/2016/09/13/uci-study-links-selfies-happiness/.

23: *smiling can lower your heart rate and stress levels:* Karen Klei-
man, "Try Some Smile Therapy," *Psychology Today*, August 1,
2012, https://www.psychologytoday.com/us/blog/isnt-what-i
-expected/201208/try-some-smile-therapy.

24: *can make you feel powerful and confident:* "Pump Up the Music—
Especially the Bass—To Make You Feel Powerful," EurekAlert!,
AAAS, August 5, 2014, https://www.eurekalert.org/pub_releases
/2014–08/sp-put080514.php.

25: *when you make yourself feel lucky:* Alexandra Ossola, "The Science
of Luck," *Popular Science*, March 17, 2015, https://www.popsci
.com/luck-real; "Keep Your Fingers Crossed: How Superstition
Improves Performance," ScienceDaily, Science News, July 14,
2010, https://www.sciencedaily.com/releases/2010/07/1007131
22846.htm.

26: *wearing a fragrance . . . can increase your self-confidence:* "The
Hidden Force of Fragrance," *Psychology Today*, November 1,
2007, last reviewed June 9, 2016, https://www.psychologytoday
.com/us/articles/200711/the-hidden-force-fragrance.

27: *wearing the color red can help you feel more confident:* Anne
Berthold, Gerhard Reese, and Judith Martin, "The Effect of Red
Color on Perceived Self-Attractiveness," *European Journal of
Social Psychology* 47, no. 5 (2017): 645–652. doi:10.1002/ejsp.2238.

27: *people wearing red:* Matthew Hutson and Tori Rodriguez, "Dress
for Success: How Clothes Influence Our Performance," *Scientific*

American, January 1, 2016, https://www.scientificamerican.com
/article/dress-for-success-how-clothes-influence-our-performance/.

2. You Can't Love Anyone Until You Love Yourself

32: *to kiss your own lips:* "Alan Watts ~ Love ~ A Dangerous Game
We Must Play." VIKTRE. February 26, 2017. https://www.viktre
.com/tai_emery/alan-watts-love-a-dangerous-game-we-must
-play. Recording of a lecture given during Watts's lifetime.

34: *being in love changes your brain:* "What Happens to Our Brain
When We're in Love?," NPR, TED Radio Hour, April 25, 2014,
https://www.npr.org/2014/04/25/301824760/what-happens-to-our
-brain-when-we-re-in-love.

35: *physical signals from the people you interact with:* "Talk Time
Featuring Dr. Stephen Porges—The Polyvagal Theory, Vocal
Prosody, Neuro-Exercises and the Face-Heart Connection,"
Dr. Rebecca Jorgensen, January 15, 2015, https://www.rebecca
jorgensen.com/talk-time-stephen-porges/.

37: *less than 4 percent of women in our society:* Amy Froneman,
"Only 4% of Women Consider Themselves Beautiful," Health24,
updated September 6, 2013, https://www.health24.com/Lifestyle
/Woman/Your-body/Only-4-of-women-consider-themselves
-beautiful-20130905.

37: *more afraid of being fat than getting cancer:* "Women's Health
Survey 2016: Unique Insights into Women's Health," Jean Hailes
for Women's Health, August 28, 2016, https://jeanhailes.org.au
/news/womens-health-survey-2016-unique-insights-into-womens
-health.

37: *her first diet at age eight:* Kelsey Miller, "Study: Most Girls Start
Dieting by Age 8," Refinery29, January 26, 2015, https://www
.refinery29.com/2015/01/81288/children-dieting-body-image
?bucketed=true&bucketing_referrer=https%3A%2F%2Fwww
.google.com%2F.

37: *fat-shamed by their peers:* Erica Goode, "Study Finds TV Alters
Fiji Girls' View of Body," *New York Times*, May 20, 1999, https://

www.nytimes.com/1999/05/20/world/study-finds-tv-alters-fiji
-girls-view-of-body.html.

45: *can have harmful effects:* Scott O. Lilienfeld and Hal Arkowitz.
"Can Positive Thinking Be Negative?," *Scientific American*, May 1,
2011, https://www.scientificamerican.com/article/can-positive
-thinking-be-negative/; Joanne V. Wood, W. Q. Elaine Perunovic,
and John W. Lee, "Positive Self-Statements," *Psychological
Science* 20, no. 7 (2009): 860–866. doi:10.1111/j.1467–9280.2009
.02370.x.

49: *here are more stats:* Coco Ballantyne, "Does Exercise Really Make
You Healthier?," *Scientific American*, January 2, 2009, https://
www.scientificamerican.com/article/does-exercise-really-make/.

50: *hard, scientific facts:* Martin Reed, "Could Masturbation Cure
Your Insomnia?," HealthCentral, May 5, 2016, https://www
.healthcentral.com/article/could-masturbation-cure-your
-insomnia; Renee Jacques, "11 Reasons You Should Be Having
More Orgasms," HuffPost, Wellness, updated December 6, 2017,
https://www.huffingtonpost.com/2013/11/05/orgasm-health
-benefits_n_4143213.html.

3. Expectations Lead to Disappointment

65: *drinking better wine than they actually were:* "Wine Tasting:
Expectations Influence Sense of Taste, Tests Show," ScienceDaily,
Science News, September 14, 2009, https://www.sciencedaily
.com/releases/2009/09/090912124050.htm.

65: *improved when they believed they'd been given an expensive drug:*
Jo Marchant, "Parkinson's Patients Trained to Respond to
Placebos," *Nature*, February 10, 2016, https://www.nature.com
/news/parkinson-s-patients-trained-to-respond-to-placebos
-1.19341.

66: *In the words of journalist and author Kathryn Schulz:* Kathryn
Schulz, On Being Wrong, March 2011, TED video, 17:15, https://
www.ted.com-talks-kathryn_schulz_on_being_wrong.

67: *existing dopamine levels take a nosedive:* David Rock, "(Not So
Great) Expectations," *Psychology Today*, November 23, 2009,

https://www.psychologytoday.com/us/blog/your-brain-work
/200911/not-so-great-expectations.

84: *Dr. Lance Dodes is a leading figure:* John Lavitt, "AA Critic Lights
Another Fire (Includes New Section)," The Fix, May 30, 2014,
https://www.thefix.com/content/14-questions-dr-lance-dodes
?page=all.

4. You Get What You Get and You Don't Get Upset

90: *the brain's ability to experience gratitude develops between the ages
of seven and ten:* Al-Jameela S. Youssef, Jeffrey J. Froh, Meagan E.
Muller, and Tara Lomas, "Measuring Gratitude in Youth:
Assessing the Psychometric Properties of Adult Gratitude Scales
in Children and Adolescents," PsycEXTRA Dataset, 2011. doi:10
.1037/e711892011–001.

92: *those who denied that sexism still exists in America:* Dina Leygerman, "You Are Not Equal. I'm Sorry," Medium, January 23, 2017,
https://www.medium.com/@dinachka82/about-your-poem-1f26a
7585a6f.

92: *according to one concordance:* James Strong, *Strong's Exhaustive
Concordance of the Bible.* Peabody, MA: Hendrickson, 2009.

93: *to keep power and control over people in this world:* Mark Y. A.
Davies, "Refusing the Hand of the Empire," One World House,
posted December 28, 2016, https://www.oneworldhouse.net/2016
/12/28/refusing-the-hand-of-the-empire/.

94: *it's all over your face:* "Written All Over Your Face: Humans
Express Four Basic Emotions Rather than Six," ScienceDaily,
Science News, February 3, 2014, https://www.sciencedaily.com
/releases/2014/02/140203113551.htm.

99: *volunteers with a fear of snakes:* Daniela Schiller, "Snakes in the
MRI Machine: A Study of Courage," *Scientific American,* July 20,
2010, https://www.scientificamerican.com/article/snakes-in-the
-mri-machine/.

101: *a unique sensation of well-being when it's satisfied:* Hans Villarica,
"Maslow 2.0: A New and Improved Recipe for Happiness," *The
Atlantic,* August 17, 2011, https://www.theatlantic.com/health

/archive/2011/08/maslow-20-a-new-and-improved-recipe-for
-happiness/243486/.

102: *people tend to be happier when the needs of others in their society
are also fulfilled:* Louis Tay and Ed Diener, "Needs and Subjective
Well-being around the World," *Journal of Personality and Social
Psychology* 101, no. 2 (2011): 354–365. doi:10.1037/a0023779.

104: A *stress-reducing practice developed in Japan:* Meeri Kim, "'Forest
Bathing' Is Latest Fitness Trend to Hit U.S.—'Where Yoga Was
30 Years Ago,'" *Washington Post*, May 17, 2016, https://www
.washingtonpost.com/news/to-your-health/wp/2016/05/17/forest-
bathing-is-latest-fitness-trend-to-hit-u-s-where-yoga-was-30
-years-ago/?utm_term=.52073adac94d.

104: *You can find good medicine in music:* Amy Novotney, "Music as
Medicine," *Monitor on Psychology* 44, no. 10, American Psychological Association, Science Watch, November 2013, https://www
.apa.org/monitor/2013/11/music.aspx.

5. Nobody Can Make You Feel Bad Without Your Permission

113: *Brain scans of adults who were bullied:* R. Douglas Fields, "Sticks
and Stones—Hurtful Words Damage the Brain," *Psychology
Today*, October 20, 2010, https://www.psychologytoday.com/us
/blog/the-new-brain/201010/sticks-and-stones-hurtful-words
-damage-the-brain.

114: *Oxytocin can nurture feelings of generosity:* Michael Kosfeld,
Markus Heinrich, Paul J. Zak, Urs Fischbacher, and Ernst Fehr,
"Oxytocin Increases Trust in Humans," *Nature* 435 (June 2005):
673–676, abstract available at https://www.nature.com/articles
/nature03701.

115: *emotions like sadness and hate can also elicit a release of oxytocin:*
Christopher Badcock, "The Dark Side of Oxytocin," *Psychology
Today*, October 24, 2016, https://www.psychologytoday.com/us
/blog/the-imprinted-brain/201610/the-dark-side-oxytocin; C. K
Dreu, L. W. De, L. Greer, G. A. Van Kleef, S. Shalvi, and M. J. J.
Handgraaf, "Oxytocin Promotes Human Ethnocentrism,"
Proceedings of the National Academy of Sciences 108, no. 4
(2011): 1262–1266. doi:10.1073/pnas.1015316108.

115: *interacting with people on social media:* Verilliance. "Social Media, Tweeting, Oxytocin and the Study That Never Was," Verilliance, August 5, 2010. Accessed July 13, 2018. https://www.verilliance .com/social-media-tweeting-oxytocin/

128: *the science on forgiveness:* Everett L. Worthington Jr., "The New Science of Forgiveness," *Greater Good Magazine*, September 1, 2004, https://www.greatergood.berkeley.edu/article/item/the _new_science_of_forgiveness.

6. Honesty Is the Best Policy

134: *The data varies, but it doesn't lie:* We do: Gad Saad, "How Often Do People Lie in Their Daily Lives?," *Psychology Today*, November 30, 2011, https://www.psychologytoday.com/us/blog/homo -consumericus/201111/how-often-do-people-lie-in-their-daily- lives; James Geary, "How to Spot a Liar," *Time*, March 13, 2000, http://content.time.com/time/world/article/0,8599,2051177,00.html; Yudhijit Bhattacharjee, "Why We Lie: The Science Behind Our Deceptive Ways," *National Geographic*, June 2017, https://www .nationalgeographic.com/magazine/2017/06/lying-hoax-false-fibs -science/; "UMass Amherst Researcher Finds Most People Lie in Everyday Conversation," UMass Amherst, News & Media Rela- tions, June 10, 2002, www.umass.edu/newsoffice/article/umass -amherst-researcher-finds-most-people-lie-everyday-conversation; Robin Lloyd, "Why We Lie," LiveScience, May 15, 2006, https:// www.livescience.com/772-lie.html; "Honesty Linked with Better Health: Study," HuffPost, Wellness, updated August 8, 2012, https://www.huffingtonpost.com/2012/08/07/honesty-healthy-lies -truth_n_1748144.html.

135: *Koko once used sign language to blame that kitten:* "Liar, Liar, Fur on Fire," Observations of Animal Behaviour, April 11, 2013, blog .nus.edu.sg/lsm1303student2013/2013/04/11/liar-liar-fur-on-fire/.

136: *Kennedy deceived the public:* "Arms Control Today." Nonprolifer- ation Benefits of India Deal Remain Elusive, Arms Control Association. Accessed July 13, 2018. https://www.armscontrol .org/act/2012_10/Reconsidering-the-Perilous-Cuban-Missile -Crisis-50-Years-Later#bernstein.

138: *Within hours of being born:* Roderick M. Kramer, "Rethinking Trust," *Harvard Business Review*, June 2009, https://www.hbr .org/2009/06/rethinking-trust.

138: *Dr. Timothy R. Levine's Truth Default Theory:* Timothy R. Levine, "Truth-Default Theory (TDT)," *Journal of Language and Social Psychology* 33, no. 4 (2014): 378–392. doi:10.1177/0261927x145 35916.

139: *means "deception, trick, scheming, intrigue":* "bull (n.3)," Online Etymology Dictionary, https://www.etymonline.com/word /bull?ref=etymonline_crossreference, accessed June 29, 2018.

141: *a study led by Dr. Robert Feldman:* Dwight B. Shepard, "The Truth Is, Most People Lie, UMass Professor Robert Feldman Says in New Book," MassLive.com, updated August 17, 2009, https://www.masslive.com/news/index.ssf/2009/08/the_truth_is _most_people_lie_u.html.

143: *consistently lying for your own benefit:* Lizette Borreli, "How Lying Affects the Human Brain: Telling Lies Desensitizes Amygdala to Dishonesty; Increases Chances of Being a Pathological Liar," *Medical Daily*, October 26, 2016, https:// www.medicaldaily.com/how-lying-affects-human-brain-telling -lies-desensitizes-amygdala-dishonesty-402310.

143: *legitimate health benefits:* "Lying Less Linked to Better Health, New Research Finds," American Psychological Association, August 4, 2012, www.apa.org/news/press/releases/2012/08/lying -less.aspx.

7. Follow Your Bliss

152: *Alain de Botton . . . observed:* Alain de Botton, "A Kinder, Gentler Philosophy of Success," TED: Ideas Worth Spreading, July 2009, https://www.ted.com/talks/alain_de_botton_a_kinder_gentler _philosophy_of_success.

154: *not just thrilled, but deeply happy:* Joseph Campbell, with Bill Moyers. *The Power of Myth* (St. Louis, MO: Turtleback Books, 2012), pp. 120, 193.

154: *"Follow Your Blisters":* Angela Hoxsey, "Follow Your Blisters," *Napa Valley Register*, December 5, 2014, https://www.napavalleyregister

.com/lifestyles/home-and-garden/columnists/angela-hoxsey /follow-your-blisters/article_a8057361-f35b-5036-ae40-a49cc0c1d 81c.html.

155: *"that life within you, all the time"*: "Follow Your Bliss," Joseph Campbell Foundation, https://www.jcf.org/about-joseph -campbell/follow-your-bliss/, accessed July 5, 2018.

155: *only* up until their cost of living is covered: D. Kahneman and A. Deaton, "High Income Improves Evaluation of Life but Not Emotional Well-being," *Proceedings of the National Academy of Sciences* 107, no. 38 (2010): 16489–16493. doi:10.1073/pnas.1011 492107.

156: *Fulfillment, meaning, and purpose in daily life vanished:* Barry Schwartz, "The Way We Think About Work Is Broken," TED: Ideas Worth Spreading, March 2014, https://www.ted.com/talks /barry_schwartz_the_way_we_think_about_work_is_broken /transcript.

157: *James Olds and Peter Milner wired up a rat:* David Lipton, "Olds & Milner, 1954: 'Reward Centers' in the Brain and Lessons for Modern Neuroscience," Stanford Neuroblog, June 10, 2013, www.web.stanford.edu/group/neurostudents/cgi-bin/wordpress /?p=3733.

158: *when a similar experiment was carried out with humans:* Christopher Bergland, "The Neuroscience of Pleasure and Addiction," *Psychology Today*, May 31, 2014, https://www.psychologytoday. com/us/blog/the-athletes-way/201405/the-neuroscience-pleasure -and-addiction.

159: *eternity is now:* Alan Watts, *Eastern Wisdom, Modern Life: Collected Talks, 1960–1969* (Novato, CA: New World Library, 2006), pp. 109–110.

159: hungry ghost: Ronald Alexander, "The Wanting Mind of Depression & Unhappiness," *Psychology Today*, June 3, 2010, https:// www.psychologytoday.com/us/blog/the-wise-open-mind/201006 /the-wanting-mind-depression-unhappiness.

162: *living life like it's a marathon, not a sprint:* Angela Lee Duckworth, "Grit: The Power of Passion and Perseverance," TED: Ideas Worth Spreading, TED Talks Education, April 2013, https://www.ted.com/talks/angela_lee_duckworth_grit_the _power_of_passion_and_perseverance/transcript?language=en.

162: *Duckworth's research:* Shana Lebowitz, "A UPenn Psychologist Says There's One Trait More Important to Success Than IQ or Talent," Business Insider, May 4, 2016, www.businessinsider.com /angela-duckworth-grit-more-important-than-iq-or-talent-2016–5.

164: *meaning the custodial staff at hospitals found in their work:* Jessica Stillman, "What You Can Learn About Job Satisfaction from a Janitor," Inc.com, June 7, 2013, https://www.inc.com /jessica-stillman/what-you-can-learn-about-career-satisfaction -from-a-hospital-janitor.html.

169: *can begin building and exercising your willpower:* Leslie Baehr, "How to Improve Willpower? Feed It," *Los Angeles Times*, November 8, 2015, http://www.latimes.com/health/la-he-willpower -20151107-story.html.

170: *changing direction when something doesn't work isn't "failing":* Astro Teller, "The Unexpected Benefit of Celebrating Failure," TED: Ideas Worth Spreading, February 2016, https://www.ted.com/talks /astro_teller_the_unexpected_benefit_of_celebrating_failure.

174: *the 1 Percent Rule:* James Altucher, "The 1% Rule for Creating All Habits," James Altucher, https://jamesaltucher.com/2015/08 /habits-one-percent/, accessed June 29, 2018.

176: *Dr. Carol Dweck ran a study:* "A Modern Stoic Clinic," Modern Stoicism, April 12, 2014, https://www.modernstoicism.com/the -philosophy-clinic-stoic-saturdays/.

176: *given an assignment that was beyond their abilities:* Pam Miracle, "Understanding a Mindset for Success," Stanford, The Clayman Institute for Gender Research, January 12, 2015, https://gender .stanford.edu/news-publications/gender-news/understanding -mindset-success.

176: *An internal report at Hewlett-Packard:* Carol S. Dweck, "Motivational Processes Affecting Learning," *American Psychologist* 41, no. 10 (1986): 1040–1048. doi:10.1037/0003–066x.41.10.1040.

8. Live Each Day Like It's Your Last

182: *The Roman emperor Marcus Aurelius wrote:* Tara Sophia Mohr, "Why Women Don't Apply for Jobs Unless They're 100% Qualified," *Harvard Business Review*, March 2, 2018. Accessed July 13, 2018. https://hbr.org/2014/08/why-women-dont-apply-for-jobs -unless-theyre-100-qualified.

182: Carpe diem *has been even more misunderstood:* Robert Hall, J. Wisniewski, and Chris Snipes, "The 5 Most Frequently Misused Proverbs," Cracked.com, February 17, 2013, https:// www.cracked.com/article_20251_the-5-most-frequently -misused-proverbs.html#ixzz2Owoxb8mB.

187: *In 2009, artist Candy Chang:* Candy Chang, "Before I Die I Want to . . . ," TED: Ideas Worth Spreading, July 2012, https://www .ted.com/talks/candy_chang_before_i_die_i_want_to.

189: *make your life personally meaningful:* "Exhibiting Artist Interview: Candy Chang," SOMArts, www.somarts.org/candychang/, accessed June 29, 2018.

191: *people who consistently keep their living spaces tidy:* Ralph Ryback, "The Powerful Psychology Behind Cleanliness," *Psychology Today*, July 11, 2016, https://www.psychologytoday.com/us/blog/the-truisms -wellness/201607/the-powerful-psychology-behind-cleanliness.

195: *will outlast our time on earth:* Ernest Becker Foundation, Theories, www.ernestbecker.org/about-becker/theories/, accessed June 29, 2018.

196: *a one in 400 trillion chance of you even existing:* Ali Binazir, "What Are the Chances of Your Coming into Being?," June 15, 2011, blogs.harvard.edu/abinazir/2011/06/15/what-are-chances -you-would-be-born/.

196: *you probably know around 600 people:* Tyler H. McCormick, Matthew J. Salganik, and Tian Zheng, "How Many People Do You Know?: Efficiently Estimating Personal Network Size," *Journal of the American Statistical Association* 105, no. 489 (2010): 59–70, https://doi.org/10.1198/jasa.2009.ap08518.

196: *you will probably meet . . . around 80,000 people:* Anna Vital, "Why We Live—Counting the People Your Life Impacts [Infographic]," Adioma, April 29, 2013, https://blog.adioma.com /counting-the-people-you-impact-infographic/.

197: *a situation you no longer have control over:* Daniel T. Gilbert and Jane E. J. Ebert, "Decisions and Revisions: The Affective Forecasting of Changeable Outcomes," *Journal of Personality and Social Psychology* 82, no. 4 (2002): 503–514, https://doi.org/10 .1037//0022–3514.82.4.503.

198: *when you* know *what needs to be done:* Neal J. Roese and Amy Summerville, "What We Regret Most . . . and Why," *Personality and Social Psychology Bulletin* 31, no. 9 (2005): 1273–1285, https://doi.org/10.1177/0146167205274693.

202: *people who made a regular practice of gratitude:* Robert A. Emmons and Michael E. McCullough, "Counting Blessings Versus Burdens: An Experimental Investigation of Gratitude and Subjective Well-Being in Daily Life," *Journal of Personality and Social Psychology* 84, no. 2 (2003): 377–389, https://doi.org /10.1037/0022–3514.84.2.377.

202: *echoed in a 2013 study:* Patrick L. Hill, Mathias Allemand, and Brent W. Roberts. "Examining the Pathways Between Gratitude and Self-Rated Physical Health Across Adulthood," *Personality and Individual Differences* 54, no. 1 (2013): 92–96, https://doi.org /10.1016/j.paid.2012.08.011.

202: *increased levels of gratitude:* Prathik Kini, Joel Wong, Sydney McInnis, Nicole Gabana, and Joshua W. Brown, "The Effects of Gratitude Expression on Neural Activity," *NeuroImage* 128: 1–10; http://doi.org/10.1016/j.neuroimage.2015.12.040; Jessica Stillman, "Gratitude Physically Changes Your Brain, New Study Says," Inc. com, January 15, 2016, https://www.inc.com/jessica-stillman /the-amazing-way-gratitude-rewires-your-brain-for-happiness .html.

203: *simply* remembering *to look for things to be grateful for:* Sonja Lyubomirsky and Kristin Layous, "How Do Simple Positive Activities Increase Well-Being?," *Current Directions in Psychological Science* 22, no. 1 (2013): 57–62, https://doi.org/10.1177/09637 21412469809.

204: thirty-two million Americans *can't read:* Valerie Strauss, "Hiding in Plain Sight: The Adult Literacy Crisis," *Washington Post*, November 1, 2016, https://www.washingtonpost.com/news /answer-sheet/wp/2016/11/01/hiding-in-plain-sight-the-adult -literacy-crisis/.

206: *further deepening their new connection and friendship:* Lisa A. Williams and Monica Y. Bartlett, "Warm Thanks: Gratitude Expression Facilitates Social Affiliation in New Relationships via Perceived Warmth," *Emotion* 15, no. 1 (2015): 1–5, https://doi .org/10.1037/emo0000017.